THE *Penelope* PROJECT

Humanities AND PUBLIC LIFE

TERESA MANGUM *&* ANNE VALK, *Series Editors*

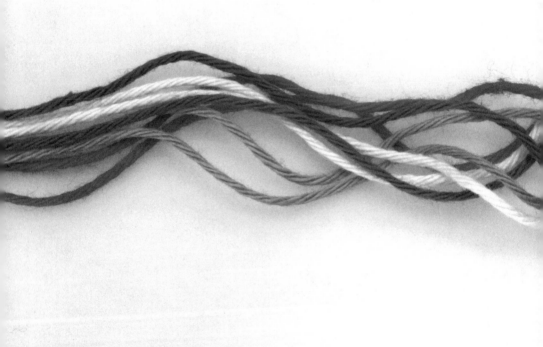

THE *Penelope* PROJECT

An Arts-Based Odyssey to Change Elder Care

EDITED BY ANNE BASTING, MAUREEN TOWEY,
AND ELLIE ROSE

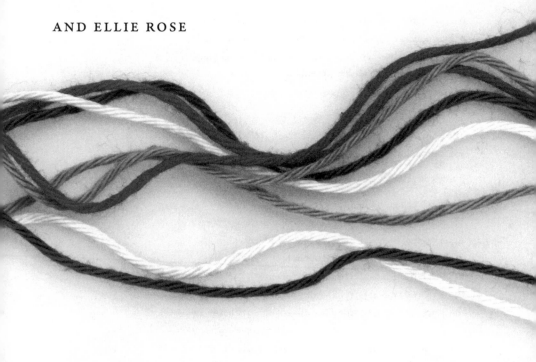

UNIVERSITY OF IOWA PRESS

Iowa City

University of Iowa Press, Iowa City 52242
Copyright © 2016 by the University of Iowa Press
www.uiowapress.org
Printed in the United States of America

Design by Richard Hendel

The University of Iowa Press is a member of Green Press Initiative
and is committed to preserving natural resources.

Printed on acid-free paper

Library of Congress Cataloging-in-Publication Data
The Penelope project : an arts-based odyssey to change elder care /
Anne Basting, Maureen Towey, and Ellie Rose, eds.
pages   cm. — (Humanities and public life)
Includes bibliographical references and index.
ISBN 978-1-60938-413-5 (pbk), ISBN 978-1-60938-414-2 (ebk)
1. Amateur theater — Wisconsin — Milwaukee.   2. Theater and older
people — Wisconsin — Milwaukee.   3. Older people — Recreation —
Wisconsin — Milwaukee.   4. Long-term care facilities — Recreational
activities — Wisconsin — Milwaukee.   I. Basting, Anne Davis,
1965-editor.   II. Towey, Maureen, editor.   III. Rose, Ellie, editor.
PN3160.A34P47   2016
792.02'220977595 — dc23   2015035744

CONTENTS

APPENDICES

SERIES EDITORS' FOREWORD

The rich collaboration documented in *The Penelope Project: An Arts-Based Odyssey to Change Elder Care* is also the backstory of the Humanities and Public Life book series. Humanities scholars have long tended to work autonomously. Anthropologists, classicists, and historians discover invaluable connections in the past that help us grasp the shaping force of the present. Scholars in literature and the arts join philosophers in offering fresh interpretations of the world around us, charting what we hope will be a wiser path to the future. That work continues. However, as that world has morphed into an almost inescapably networked landscape, we humanities scholars find ourselves working in much closer proximity to the audiences to whom we used to write from a distance.

While the resulting connections often remain virtual, many scholars and artists have embraced new opportunities to work not only in a more public fashion but with public partners. These partners include natural allies we often call the "public humanities"—state humanities councils, historical societies, libraries, museums, and performances venues—but also surprising partners from prisons to housing projects, from retirement communities to restored prairies. Suddenly, artists and scholars find themselves living as well as learning the arts and humanities. These are the stories between the covers of the books in our series.

We—the coeditors—met thanks to the consortium Imagining America: Artists and Scholars in Public Life. Each year the annual conference brings together artists and scholars whose groundbreaking projects position the humanities and arts at the core of efforts to better the communities we share. Challenged and inspired by the surprising sites and partners that artists and scholars find when they plunge into public life, we wanted to ensure that their stories would have the greatest influence possible. How, we asked ourselves, could the astonishing projects we kept encountering at Imagining America and across the country be brought to classrooms and communities across the country?

We are delighted that Imagining America has stepped into that breach by creating a rigorously reviewed online journal, *PUBLIC*, to document the power of engaged arts and scholarship. Our book series, Humanities and Pub-

lic Life, takes another leap by providing publicly engaged artists and humanists greater space to share and reflect upon large and complicated projects
that unfold over time. More often than not the achievements and impact of
such collaborations are unexpected, myriad, ongoing, and the best of what
the humanities can be—life-changing.

That is certainly the case with the Penelope Project, chronicled here.
It involved theatre scholars and students at the University of Wisconsin–
Milwaukee, led by Anne Basting and partners at Luther Manor (a retirement community) and Sojourn Theatre company. Basting's coeditors rep-
resent just two of the overlapping communities woven together through
the Penelope Project. Ellie Rose is a visual artist and a specialist in dementia
care who oversaw Adult Day Services at the Luther Manor retirement community, and Maureen Towey directs performance events and is an ensemble
member of Sojourn Theatre.

What connects the artists, designers, social scientists, and humanities
scholars who we hope will find a published home in our series is their un-
shakeable optimism in what publicly engaged artists and scholars have to
contribute. We share their conviction that through engaged practices, the
arts and humanities can simultaneously strengthen our educational system,
generate deeper knowledge of our world and peoples' responses to it across
time and space, and genuinely benefit our communities. The projects we have
seen already have the potential to inspire a revolution in what we *do* with the
humanities and what the humanities can do for us—as students, scholars,
and members of varied and overlapping communities.

The authors of our books take the word "engagement" seriously. Imagining America's definition provides a compass:

> *Publicly Engaged Scholarship* is defined by partnerships of university
> knowledge and resources with those of the public and private sectors
> to enrich scholarship, research, creative activity, and public knowledge;
> enhance curriculum, teaching and learning; prepare educated, engaged
> citizens; strengthen democratic values and civic responsibility; address
> and help solve critical social problems; and contribute to the public
> good. (http://imaginingamerica.org/about/our-mission/)

While not all of the projects in our series involve colleges and universities, our long-term goal is to capture the boundless capacity of culture and
cultural practice to animate the values, responsibilities, and lifelong learning
that genuine democracy demands.

Like "engagement," the word "humanities" can inspire more confusion than clarity. Yet the humanities have long been acknowledged as fundamental to public life in the United States—even when economic anxieties tempt politicians to argue that the arts and humanities are peripheral rather than profoundly necessary to maintain a good society. The National Endowment for the Humanities (NEH), founded in 1965, surveys the many fields of knowledge that form our heritage and enable us to imagine our future. Again, a definition is worth quoting in full:

> The term "humanities" includes, but is not limited to, the study and interpretation of the following: language, both modern and classical; linguistics; literature; history; jurisprudence; philosophy; archaeology; comparative religion; ethics; the history, criticism and theory of the arts; those aspects of social sciences which have humanistic content and employ humanistic methods; and the study and application of the humanities to the human environment with particular attention to reflecting our diverse heritage, traditions, and history and to the relevance of the humanities to the current conditions of national life. (http://www.neh.gov/about)

We expect to find examples of publicly engaged scholarship embedded in all of these disciplines to be included in this series.

Collectively, the series will make visible an emerging third space that overlaps, integrates, animates, and expands learning through collective commitment to the greater good of communities—local, national, and global as well as past, present, and future. This realm, and the desire to foster it, is not new. The NEH has long attempted to bridge the gap between the academic humanities and public humanities—that is, between colleges and universities, on one hand, and libraries, museums, performance spaces, and state humanities councils, on the other. Until recently these bridges tended to be on paths unfamiliar to colleges and universities. Now new maps are being drawn. The NEH's "Common Good" initiative challenges humanists "to bring the humanities into the public square and foster innovative ways to make scholarship relevant to contemporary issues." Through narrative, reflection, assessment, and example, the authors in our series can help to surface that public character and potential of the humanities to enrich communities across the country.

The power of publicly engaged artists and scholars to galvanize learning through collaboration with community partners brings us back to Penelope Project.

In the coming decades, more and more of us will find ourselves retiring, accommodating to changes our society considers losses, and negotiating a sense of our long-held identities with the often cruel imposition of assumptions about old age by people around us. What do the humanities have to do with growing old?

One of the driving interests in Basting's scholarly and creative work and her longtime collaboration with Luther Manor is a simple, overwhelming question one faces when working with people suffering from dementia: How do we communicate with someone who no longer has memory? What she has learned, in part through her work with Rose and Towey, is that even without memory, people can participate in storytelling and performance. But the forms of storytelling familiar to most of us are inadequate to the collective, fragmentary, and fading narratives created by those without memory.

Basting's first major project, TimeSlips, invited students, caretakers, family members, actors, and people with memory loss to experience narratives of Alzheimer's patients from inside their point of view. The Penelope Project goes even further by drawing together the shared expertise of colleagues at Luther Manor, members of the extraordinary Sojourn Theatre, faculty and students from the University of Wisconsin–Milwaukee, and older people themselves to stage a play—*Finding Penelope*.

Through endless planning and patient engagement with local agencies, care facilities, student programs, photographers, and filmmakers, the group discovered material for their performance while also transforming the lives of every participant. So often we focus on the "product" of one endeavor or another; *Finding Penelope* is creativity and imagination in action. Rooted in classical mythology and collaborative performance, the Penelope Project weaves imagery; symbolic action; fragments of sound, color, and events; collaborators; and viewers into an uncannily beautiful expression of empathy with and faith in the human spirit across the generations.

This early book in our series offers new worlds of possibility to faculty members and students from disciplines as seemingly distant as geriatrics and classics, public health and performing arts, social work and history. We believe this book will also inspire people whose lives and careers in retirement communities and nursing facilities are dedicated to supporting a joyful late life. We hope that, whatever your talents and wherever you are situated in your work and community, this book will convince you that we all have life-affirming roles to play as committed citizens who believe we can create a better world together through engaged and collaborative arts, culture, and education.

We warmly thank the many participants in the Penelope Project for sharing their story with us so that we can share it with you.

TERESA MANGUM AND ANNE VALK
Humanities and Public Life, Series Editors

FOREWORD

This is a "performative" book: it does what it describes. Spoken by many voices telling a story of many parts, and each part with many participants, its vision of collaboration and community is enacted in the collaborative form taken by the book itself. The Penelope Project, and its book, create a world in which no one is left out. But this book is not an account of some utopian dream. It is also a practical manual, a manual of practice, describing the steps taken by a set of unlikely partners — university students and their teachers, a theatre company, and a nursing home along with its residents and staff.

The project culminated in the creation of a play, *Finding Penelope*. The more theatre-oriented reader may think that putting on a show as a community project was the singular motive of the labor that came before. But the book reveals longer-term goals. The Penelope Project was an attempt to undo entrenched social disregard of the old, to transform routine institutional elder care, and to break through the fear of advanced age often experienced by the young.

Taking place over a two-year period, from 2009 to 2011, the Penelope Project began with an agreement among three principal collaborators: the Milwaukee-based theatre professor, arts activist, and advocate for the aged, Anne Davis Basting; the Luther Manor retirement community, also in Milwaukee; and the Sojourn Theatre company, known for devising community theatre pieces based on extensive community research. Basting proposed, and Luther Manor and Sojourn agreed to engage in, a social and theatre experiment of a kind that had never been tried before. Basting is a professor in the University of Wisconsin–Milwaukee Department of Theatre and was the founding director of the university's Center for Age and Community from 2003 until 2013. Luther Manor runs a vast campus of senior services, including a nursing home and a retirement residence. The decision to work together on an arts project sustained over two years would potentially disrupt every well-oiled routine of this fifty-year-old highly respected institution, while, on Basting's end, students might not want to spend a term off-campus at a nursing home interviewing old people and seeking responses to the story of the faithful wife Penelope in the *Odyssey*. Even Sojourn Theatre would be moving beyond its experience by working with nursing home residents, many with dementia.

The reader will be struck by the different languages these three collaborating communities — the eldercare, the academic, and the theatrical — speak, and presumably spoke to each other, in the two years of work on the project. For theatre people, no clear distinction may come to mind when a nursing home director speaks of the difference between "institution-centered" and "person-centered" care. Arts language such as "applied theatre," "devised theatre," and "civic practice" (related to the visual art world's "social practice") may be mysterious to those with a nursing or social work background. And did the families of the university students involved in the project understand that their children were getting course credit for studying "service learning," "public scholarship," and "community engagement"? "Engagement" is a word on the lips of all three communities in this project: did it have the same meaning in each of their worlds?

As is clear from her presence in the dialogues of all three communities spoken in this book, Anne Davis Basting is the prime mover and visionary behind the Penelope Project. She is by now a — perhaps *the* — leading theorist/practitioner in the United States working to enliven the quality of life for the elderly, especially those with dementia, through the arts. She has conducted multiyear projects, including the storytelling project "TimeSlips" and the mixed media "Islands of Milwaukee" (another project with Sojourn Theatre) designed to raise community awareness about the physical isolation of homebound elderly. It is beyond the scope of this writing to describe these projects here, but they have a robust presence online. What links all Basting's projects is their theatrical imagination.

Readers might well ask, why theatre? Granted, it is fun to put on a show, but why should theatre occupy such a privileged place in the broad field of community organization and geriatrics that this book describes? Why would a professor of theatre find her way to that particular use of her gifts? To this writer, admittedly a theatre person, the answer lies in the nature of theatre itself.

When Basting wrote her doctoral dissertation on the representation of age on the Broadway stage, which became her first book, *Stages of Age*, she was warned by her professors that she would never get a job. Theatre departments were not looking for specialists in age, they told her. But from a wider point of view, it is clear that underlying the Penelope Project was the communitarian vision that the making of theatre itself represents. Theatre forges a bond unlike any other, tying its makers to each other and their theatre to its community. Thus what may look like a puzzling leap from academic theatre into community service was a visionary extension of Basting's earliest interest.

Over the two years of the project, new community feeling sprouted in the environment of the Penelope Project. Students, originally afraid of old people, began to bond with them. Residents of the Luther Manor assisted living complex ventured into the adjacent nursing home for the first time. Some of them were cast in leading roles and performed alongside the professional Sojourn actors. And when the play was finally mounted, the general public was welcomed into the nursing home, which now opened itself as a performance venue. To quote a famous line from Ibsen's play *Hedda Gabler*, "People don't do such things."

No example in the Penelope work better describes this theatrical ideal of inclusivity than the weaving. Penelope, so the myth goes, managed for years to forestall the one hundred some suitors who sought her hand and plagued her palace until such time as she would complete the weaving of her father-in-law's funeral shroud. Yet every night she secretly ripped out the weaving of the day, placating the suitors while at the same time deceiving them. In that way she stayed true to her absent husband Odysseus. The Penelope play makers found a way to "weave" the weaving motif into the Milwaukee experiment that solved a traffic problem, a design problem, and, perhaps most of all, an inclusion problem. The latter was the resolution to an issue that troubled Basting and her colleagues: How could they sweep Luther Manor's many frail residents and their staff attendants into a sense of identification with a sustained, larger project? (This is the "beyond Bingo" problem that troubles many in the geriatric care field: how to get beyond daily activities to more sustained goals.)

The play, *Finding Penelope*, used a variety of spaces in Luther Manor as its set, cleverly layering the classical sites of the ancient Greek story over the public rooms of the nursing home. Every scene location was both everyday and nontheatrical, and at the same time a place of the mythic imagination. The tale of the faithful Penelope, here a "heroine of waiting," was told as a double journey of reunion. One, as in the *Odyssey*, was the reunion of Penelope with her husband; the other was her reconciliation with a devised character, a daughter, who had abandoned her mother to the nursing home, staying away out of fear and anticipated disgust. The journey into the palace/

nursing home and toward the site of these twin recognition scenes was taken by the audience as well, who traversed a long course of corridors and stairways that led into the home's working space.

The designer of Sojourn Theatre, Shannon Scrofano, hit upon the idea of having the residents of Luther Manor, many confined to wheelchairs and not robust enough to participate as chorus in the play, create what became a half-mile skein of colorful weaving, a project that took months to achieve. Luther Manor's Ellie Rose figured out that it could be made by the residents, together with the staff, out of colorful ribbons of fabric and plastic six-pack strips, which come not in sixes but in continuous rolls. "Weaving" the cloth strips in and out through the lid-size openings was just right for older hands. The completed skein was then hung along the walls and up the stairs to keep the audience from straying off limits.

This design element was a stroke of genius, resonating, as good theatre always does, with many lines of meaning. The project showed the value and beauty of objects normally disregarded and thrown away—rags, six-pack plastics—pointing of course to the value of people with dementia who are sometimes treated as throwaways themselves; it involved the entire community of residents and caretakers in a sustained joint project that, like making theatre itself, had a goal beyond individual entertainment or gratification. In this sly way, even the famous beer-making industry of Milwaukee made a cameo appearance, reminding the audience that we were not only in a fictive universe but in the home of Blatz, Pabst, and Miller.

This writer was privileged to perform a small role in the carrying out of what I might call the Penelope mandate. As the introductory material in the book makes clear, funding for Penelope came from sources as diverse as its makers. A major grant required documentation of the project's results. Thus a "think tank" of diverse professionals was invited to see a performance, with each invitee assigned a response from his or her own field of expertise, to be offered in a separate day of analysis, responses that in turn were to be recorded and transcribed. Brought to Milwaukee from different cities and institutions, many in this group met for the first time on the bus transporting us to the nursing home.

We began as strangers and ended as intimates, a transformation that took no longer than the performance itself. After following *Finding Penelope* through the nursing home to the great ingathering at its end in the auditorium and chapel, the think tank members stumbled out to the reception hall where we had begun our journey ninety minutes earlier. Some of us were sobbing, and all of us were surprised at the power of our responses. We had been through something together. We gathered in our own corner of the hall. Words tumbled out about our parents' illnesses and deaths, our relationships with our children, about grief and mourning and fear of aging and our admiration for the work. As a professional theatre critic, I struggled for words that would express the difference between a mere theatrical experience, as profound as such an experience can occasionally be, and this just-past experience of immersion in a place where the very "setting" and so many of the resident performers performed themselves. We came as designated outsiders, but like everyone else involved with the Penelope Project, we were not to be left out.

Theorists of the theatre sometimes describe it as a model, or a "scale model," of human experience. One recalls the famous scene in Ingmar Bergman's *Fanny and Alexander* in which the leader of the theatrical family toasts the "little world" of the theatre as one that nonetheless embraces and contains the "big world" of reality. The Penelope Project reversed this relationship. Illness, death, and grief were not merely performed; they were ever present. Indeed, students and actors more than once arrived at the home to find that a participant in the play's chorus had died overnight. Here the reality of the big world was itself the frame, yet was made more legible, bearable, and beautiful, by theatre.

ELINOR FUCHS
Yale School of Drama
July 2015

INTRODUCTION: THIS BOOK, THIS STORY
Anne Basting

> *Penelope was an adventure of an unknown destiny.*
> —*Cheryl Schmitz, Director of Volunteer Services, Luther Manor*

This book tells the story of the Penelope Project. Penelope, as the collaborators simply called it, was a multiyear effort to engage a long-term care community in a retelling of Homer's *Odyssey* from the perspective of Penelope — the queen of Ithaca, cunning and courageous wife of Odysseus, and hero who never left home.

Our vision was to bring together university arts students and professional artists together with a long-term care community to collaboratively create a work of art that could transform the community into a place of storytelling and meaning-making. The core collaborative partners in Penelope were Sojourn Theatre, a professional theatre company; University of Wisconsin–Milwaukee's Center on Age & Community and the Department of Theatre; and Luther Manor, a continuing care retirement community.

Together, our unified objective was to improve the quality of life of everyone who lives, works, and visits Luther Manor. The partners knew at the outset of Penelope that we were trying to do something unusual and challenging on all fronts of the collaboration. Students don't rush to sign up for community-engaged courses in long-term care settings. Care providers aren't eager to add long-range, intensive collaboration and art-making to their already overloaded schedules. Artists don't typically stage professional performances (with paying audiences) inside of the second-most regulated industry in the United States (next to nuclear power). What kind of artistic freedom might be possible in such an environment? Could we do it? We wondered that every day — right up to the very last performance.

The artists and educators involved in this project have years of experience in community-engaged arts practice. My work with TimeSlips Creative Storytelling and Sojourn's work in civic performance are featured in many books in the field. But even we felt like we were breaking ground with this ambitious project. We looked for models — and for writing that captured the breadth of large-scale, multi-partnered, cross-sector projects. We found little to guide us. We hope this book fills that gap—supplying a full documentation of a large-scale project from start to finish.

Throughout this book, we share stories of what unfolded and what we learned on this most adventurous of journeys. This is not a "how-to" manual. Because Penelope was built of the unique assets of the collaborators, we don't imagine anyone will replicate exactly what we did. But we believe that our experiences can be helpful to inform those who strive for similar goals: (1) for artists who aim to make meaningful art in cross-sector partnerships; (2) for students who desire meaningful experiences in engaged classroom settings and learning more about complex, community-engaged arts practice; and (3) for those working to transform long-term care into the kind of place that supports and nurtures rather than maintains or harms the human psyche. From beginning to end, we thoroughly documented the project. We hope this book provides a rare window into phases of projects like Penelope that are seldom brought to light—funding, conceptualization, partnership development, and evaluation. We include some of the tools we developed throughout the project in the appendix in the hopes that they might be useful to others to adapt to their own situations and settings.

Our aim and challenge in telling the story of Penelope is to reflect, in book form, the intensely collaborative and iterative nature of the project. The process of planning and writing the book gave us a chance to extend the partnerships born and solidified in the course of creating the project itself. We, the editors and our Penelope collaborators, collectively decided how best to structure the book. The multivoiced quality of the Penelope Project, then, manifests itself in the multivoiced structure of the book. Essays roughly follow the evolution of the project from beginning to end. Where there are aberrations in chronology, we will try to orient you on your journey through the story of the project. The essays are written from a variety of viewpoints— older participants, students, artists, and care providers. Many of the essays are written in dialogue, mirroring how the project evolved. We selected editors from each core partner organization, and they bore the responsibility of ensuring their members were engaged and appropriately represented in the book-writing process. Maureen Towey, who directed the culminating *Finding Penelope* play, represents the artists' perspective for Sojourn Theatre. Ellie Rose is the core editor for the Luther Manor staff/resident/volunteer perspective. Ellie also happens to be trained as an artist. Anne Basting is also a hybrid voice—representing the faculty/student perspective and also serving as the playwright and overall project coordinator. Her extensive experience working in partnership with long-term care gives her a unique foothold in all three worlds.

Penelope was designed to be an *accessible* project. We aimed for all activities to be accessible to people with cognitive and/or physical disabilities so that they were included as full participants. This meant that we used many formats in the project — movement, poetry, visual art — that go beyond text and engage people with a variety of life experiences and learning styles. To mirror that process, throughout the book we have inserted a story of Penelope told through images. They are meant to stand alone but also roughly correspond to the timeline relayed by the essays. We also direct readers to our website (www.thepenelopeproject.com) for more visuals and video footage of Penelope. A fifty-two-minute documentary is also available for purchase on the site.

Finally, all throughout Penelope, we worked to use and clarify language to ensure that everyone entering the project felt embraced and capable of growing with it. For example, we use the words "devising" and "site-specific work" to define the process and methodology used by Sojourn Theatre artists. We also use terms like "person-centered care" to describe the underlying value system the project promotes for changing long-term care. Words like "writer" and "artist" mean different things to Luther Manor staff and residents; students at University of Wisconsin–Milwaukee's Peck School of the Arts; and Sojourn ensemble members. Words like "Alzheimer's" can strike an abstract fear or be a lived reality, depending on your context. One of our guidelines in Penelope was that people could ask "HUH?" at any point — signaling a need for clarification of terminology. No judgment. Just clarification. "What do you mean when you use that word?" We apply that guideline to this book as well, and we strive throughout to use a language that is accessible — to older adults; artists from a range of fields; staff at any level; students and faculty from any discipline. To help achieve this goal we define terms along the way and provide additional clarity with examples in a terminology appendix.

The book is organized into five parts that generally follow the chronology of the project. Part one addresses the overarching landscape of the multiple fields on which the three partnering organizations play — education; the arts; and long-term care. These essays explore where Penelope fits into the larger fields. Part two examines how we took our first steps in developing Penelope. Where did the ideas come from? How were the partnerships forged and nourished? Part three shares some of our challenges and hard-fought discoveries along the way. Part four looks to the project's rewards and successes.

Finally, part five looks at the impact and evolution of the project. What happened after the final performance? Can we say there was lasting impact? How do we know?

In the ancient stories, Penelope the queen of Ithaca was a weaver. She wove to share companionship with her maids. She wove to put off the advances of the 108 suitors who took over her home and pressured her to remarry. Weaving—as narrative, as memory—became a central metaphor in Penelope, one that is reflected here in the very structure of the essays and the book. This project, built by anyone who joined and committed to it, was itself a multi-voiced weaving. It was a long, challenging process of clarifying and entwining the goals, procedures, and languages of three different fields/systems. It was a rich, rewarding, and frustrating process of constantly inviting people to join us as collaborators. We hope this book continues that effort—earnestly inviting people from very different fields and life experiences to learn along with us.

In its original form, Greek epic poetry was made new each time singers added their own interpretations. The oldest singers were the most revered, and they incorporated the additions and embellishments of singers before them. Many of the participants in Penelope have passed away; their voices are now echoes, finding their way to the readers only through the memories of the many writers. We hope our "singing" of these words does them justice.

WHO WAS PENELOPE? YOU ASK

Most commonly, Penelope is known as the wife of Odysseus in the ancient epic the *Odyssey*. But she was so much more . . .

When Penelope was newly married and a new mother, Odysseus (king of Ithaca) was forced to fight in the Trojan War. The war lasted for ten years. But as soldiers began to come back home, Penelope's husband was not among them. Stories of his bravery came back with the returning soldiers, but Odysseus did not. As years passed, "suitors," or the marriageable men of Ithaca and nearby kingdoms, began to arrive to court Penelope. Eventually 108 of them filled her castle, killing and eating Ithaca's herds and generally abusing the Greek codes of hospitality.

Penelope raised their son, Telemachus, alone and protected him from the suitors. She put off choosing a new husband by promising to pick one of the suitors when she finished weaving a funeral shroud for her father-in-law, Laertes. All day long she would weave with her maids. And at night, they would unravel what they had woven. Eventually, the suitors learned of her deception and they renewed their pressure on her to choose among them.

One day a stranger appears — an old beggar, bent and broken. The suitors mock and abuse him, again breaking Greek codes of hospitality and the imperative to "welcome the stranger." In contrast, Penelope welcomes him, asking him for stories he might have heard of her dear husband. This old beggar is Odysseus, disguised by the goddess Athena to keep him safe from the suitors in his own home. Penelope asks him what he thinks of her plan to select a suitor by choosing the one who can string Odysseus' bow and shoot an arrow through twelve axe handles. The old beggar quickly approves — as he knows that he is the only one who can do this.

⌢‿

Eurycleia is Penelope's most trusted maid and was Odysseus' nurse maid when he was a boy. When she gives Odysseus a footbath, she recognizes a scar on his leg and discovers the truth — that after twenty years, Penelope's husband has returned. Odysseus demands that she keep his secret to protect all their lives. Odysseus and his son, Telemachus (who also knows the truth), plot to kill all the suitors at the great banquet that evening, which, with the help of Athena, they do handily.

Even after Odysseus strings his own bow and kills all 108 suitors, Penelope is cautious. She does not recognize Odysseus and is reluctant to open her heart again after so many years. She devises one last test—demanding that her marriage bed be removed from her bedroom. Odysseus becomes irate—he built that bed from a living olive tree—it can't be moved! With this, our cautious and cunning Penelope is at last convinced that Odysseus has come home.

EXCERPT FROM *Finding Penelope,* SCENE 1

Anne Basting

The Penelope Project culminated in an original play, crafted from the Penelope story and the months of engagement with the staff, volunteers, and residents at Luther Manor retirement community. In it we built parallel journeys in the mythic realms of the *Odyssey* and the real-life setting of Luther Manor. Odysseus arrives at home (disguised as a beggar) after twenty years, with hopes that Penelope will recognize and welcome him home. Mira, a fictional "bad daughter," arrives at Luther Manor to visit her mother for the first time in twenty years — also hoping that her mother will recognize and welcome her. Together, they search to find their Penelope. You will find excerpts from *Finding Penelope* throughout the book.

Scene 1: On the story of Penelope

OLD BEGGAR
Excuse me, dear lady — I might be of service here. I know the tale quite well.
I believe it starts something like —
"Sing to me of the MAN, Muse, the MAN of twists and turns
driven time and again off course, once he had plundered
the hallowed heights of Troy."

OLD NURSE
No. I don't think so — I think our story goes something like:
"Sing to me oh Muse, of the WOMAN who planted her feet
into the rocky hills of Ithaca,
driven time and again to forget the forward movement of time
and believe, time and again, in a hazy memory of a love profound."

OLD BEGGAR
I'm afraid I know it all too well — it continues:
"Many cities of men he saw and learned their minds,
many pains he suffered, heartsick on the open sea,
fighting to save his life and bring his comrades home."

OLD NURSE
No dear, actually — who are you?

OLD BEGGAR

No one of importance, gentle lady.

OLD NURSE reads his nametag.

OLD NURSE

Old Beggar? I am OLD Nurse and I know old. You? You don't look so old.

OLD BEGGAR

I'm older by the second.

OLD NURSE

Aren't we all, my friend! But I warn you kindly *Old* Beggar, you don't want
to test my Homer. The words of the *Odyssey* have pulsed through these
veins for centuries . . . and now I've made them my own. HERE is how THIS
story goes —
(*as though reading from the* Odyssey) "Many days, months and years SHE
saw turn
Days months and years
Many pains she suffered, fighting to raise a son — alone
fighting to guide a kingdom without a king.
She would wait.
She would weave.
She would win.
days, months and years
SHE would trick them all
and never settle for less than her dignity. Her love, profound."

OLD BEGGAR

I see — it is indeed her story. I'm eager to hear more.

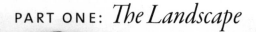

> *Penelope is more than a name. It goes beyond the remembrance of an*
> *artfully poignant play. It was a springboard into what achievements await*
> *beyond* Penelope. *As long there are minds open to imaginative cultivation,*
> *there will be* Penelope.
> —*Rusty Tym, resident, Luther Manor*

This section explores the context for the Penelope Project from the perspective of our multiple partners—long-term care, theatre-making/art, and higher education. What was the state of the field at the time the project began? What landscape did the Penelope Project step into, and what promise did it hold?

Kirsten Jacobs is trained as an artist, holds an MSW, and is education development manager for Leading Age, a membership organization for nonprofit aging-services providers. Jacobs shares her perspective on the state of "activities" in long-term care and the culture change movement that Penelope exemplified. In the old top-down approach, directors of activities assembled older adults into large groups and coordinated activities like exercise groups, bingo and sing-alongs, or, even more passively, listening to people read or to guest artists play music or sing. In the new model, directors of activities are giving way to people who coordinate elder interests and create opportunities for them to create their own programming and art.

Michael Rohd, artistic director of Sojourn Theatre and director of the Center for Performance and Civic Practice, defines the rapidly growing and shifting terrain of civic efforts in the arts and how Penelope fits into that terrain. Rather than commenting on life from galleries and theatres, Rohd is part of a growing effort to integrate artists into partnerships in the civic realm—with parks systems, with local government, with school systems. Civically engaged performances might take place in traditional theatre spaces, but they might also be staged where the performance can directly engage the desired audience—in city council chambers, schools, parks, or even long-term care settings.

Jan Cohen-Cruz, an internationally recognized expert in performance and community engagement, positions Penelope in the scope of that work with a particular focus on student engagement. Research increasingly suggests that students who participate in engaged classrooms—learning "in the field"—have a deeper grasp of the material. Imagining America, an organization that Cohen-Cruz directed for several years, supports efforts to foster engaged learning and research in the arts, humanities, and design fields.

THE CURRENT LANDSCAPE OF ACTIVITIES/
PROGRAMMING IN LONG-TERM CARE
Kirsten M. Jacobs

As a child, I often found myself performing in nursing homes with my dance or violin classes. Whether I was playing "Twinkle, Twinkle" on my half-size violin or tap dancing on the linoleum floors, I was among the children who are often paraded through nursing home hallways in hopes of brightening the lives of those who live there.

I don't remember a lot about those visits, but I do remember feeling a bit uncomfortable and afraid. The smells, sights, and sounds were all unfamiliar and somewhat unpleasant to my childhood self. I remember what I now would describe as vacant looks on the faces of some of the older adults. And I remember the hospital-like space. The hallways were long and the lighting was harsh.

About twenty years later, I once again found myself being led down a nursing home hallway, but this time in Wauwatosa, Wisconsin, and the experience was very different. As an audience member of *Finding Penelope*, I had the chance to travel through the Luther Manor community and witness the magic of the Penelope Project collaboration.

To me, the Penelope Project is an example of the ways the aging-services field and long-term care activities have evolved in recent years. Fortunately, many nursing homes are very different than they were twenty or thirty years ago. The Penelope Project is one manifestation of that evolution.

CULTURE CHANGE
About the time my childhood self was performing in nursing homes, a grassroots movement to radically change long-term care was just emerging. That movement was dubbed the culture change movement and refers to a shift away from a medical model of care. Rather than spaces and days designed to accommodate the needs of an institution, nursing home environments and schedules (or lack of schedules) are designed to accommodate the lives of those who live and work there. The terms "culture change," "person-centered care," "person-directed," and "relationship-centered care" all refer to this transformation from a medical model to a more homelike model.

Culture change is a philosophy, but there are a host of practical implications, too. Long-term care settings (like nursing and assisted living communities) are changing language, routines, activities, physical design, dining, and bathing and care practices. For example, rather than scheduling breakfast at 8:00 a.m. and waking residents at 6:00 a.m., a person-centered approach invites residents to rise when they wake and to eat what they want, when they want. People are at the heart of the culture change movement, and the place they live is their home.

To ensure the daily experience of living in a long-term care community reflects residents' likes and dislikes, great effort is made to really know them. Staff members are encouraged to spend time with residents and understand the whole person, rather than just knowing a collection of diagnoses and care needs.

This came to life recently at one West Coast organization that recruited volunteers to sit with health center (nursing home) residents to document their stories, reflections, and anecdotes. The health center residents, many of whom had dementia, shared stories about travel, past jobs, and loves. The stories were carefully documented in the words of the elders. Then, one evening, volunteers performed the vignettes for a packed house of residents, family members, and community members. The residents who participated enjoyed the experience of being heard and celebrated while staff and community members all marveled at how many new things they learned about each resident.

As evidenced by the story above, the field of "activities" (social and physical programming in long-term care) has benefitted immensely from the person-centered effort to know the people who live in nursing homes. But it's not difficult to conjure images of traditional activities programs of the past. Admittedly some nursing homes continue to plan and facilitate activities just as they did twenty years ago. In those settings, residents participate in regimented activities like bingo, birthday parties, and coffee talk. Those activities may not reflect resident preferences or interests and are often very predictable. The old paradigm assumes less capacity and keeps residents in the role of recipient rather than participant. Elders receive care and entertainment but often aren't invited to contribute, engage, or interact.

As the approach to activities in long-term care evolves, new terminology is being used to describe the daily life of the organization. Some organizations have replaced the word "activities" with "life enrichment," "wellness," "quality of life," or "life engagement." Life enrichment is currently the most common alternative to "activities," but all the terms are intended to suggest more meaningful engagement and a higher level of participation on the part of the elders.

In long-term care settings that embrace culture change, life enrichment is a way of life rather than just a program. Elders are invited to participate in daily tasks, just as they did in their own homes. So rather than special event preparation happening behind the scenes, elders might envision the event, make the decorations, prepare some of the food, and welcome the guests.

In 2006, the Centers for Medicare and Medicaid Services (CMS), the federal body that governs activities in nursing homes, affirmed the importance of culture change. CMS implemented new guidelines that state that "the facility must provide for an ongoing program of activities designed to meet, in accordance with the comprehensive assessment, the interests and the physical, mental, and psychosocial well-being of each resident" (DHHS 2006). Suddenly, nursing homes were required to tailor their activities programs to the residents living within their community. With this, activities programs that hadn't yet implemented person-centered care had to make a change. Culture change is still implemented to varying degrees across the country, but the shift in regulations pushed most organizations to think more intentionally about the ways they implement person-centered care within the nursing home environment (and often beyond).

WELLNESS

Over the past ten years, providers of aging services are increasingly striving to find ways to help both residents and employees achieve overall wellness. Many variables influenced this trend, including health care reform and a national conversation about prevention of chronic diseases and about overall well-being.

While every organization defines wellness differently, the concept generally incorporates the following dimensions: emotional, intellectual, physical, vocational, social, and spiritual. Wellness is about achieving holistic well-being for every individual. Traditionally, a nursing home might have focused primarily on physical health by administering medications, offering a healthy diet, and encouraging occasional exercise. An organization that embraces a wellness model focuses on every dimension of wellness, understanding that they are all intrinsically connected. Each element is considered equally as important as the next.

Some organizations are blending the dimensions of wellness into existing activities programs, while others are completely replacing activities with a holistic wellness program. There's huge variation from one organization to the next, but most programs strive to help elders achieve individual well-being, regardless of age or physical limitations. That means that all individuals, including those living in long-term care or approaching the end of their lives, are assumed to have the capacity to learn and grow in all dimensions of life.

The Penelope Project invited residents to participate in discussion groups, movement exercises, visual art making, music making, and storytelling. Together, the project addressed every element of holistic wellness. Engaging with other residents, university students, actors, and community members addressed social and emotional wellness. Participating in movement exercises enhanced physical well-being. Learning about the *Odyssey* through discussion groups, storytelling, and other projects provided opportunities for intellectual growth. Preparing for the *Finding Penelope* production by helping with set design contributed to vocational wellness. Aspects of the play, like the chorus' "Welcome Dance" ("My heart is open to you, my soul/spirit welcomes you"), illustrated that spiritual well-being doesn't happen only in Bible study. The Penelope Project is one of many examples of long-term care settings finding big ways to incorporate all the dimensions of wellness into the daily lives of those who live there.

ARTS AND CREATIVITY

Arts and crafts have traditionally been a part of long-term care activities, but organizations now go well beyond an occasional craft project. With steadily growing evidence to support the value of the arts and creativity in the lives of elders, long-term care organizations are incorporating varied opportunities into their life enrichment programs.

One East Coast organization opened its building to the greater community by offering a space for professional artists and musicians to store their supplies and instruments in exchange for conducting art classes for residents. In other organizations, residents participate in dance classes that incorporate storytelling and poetry. Some organizations use the techniques of improvisation to both train staff and engage elders. Whether it is storytelling, dancing, or art-making, long-term care settings are striving to make the arts accessible to all residents, including those with physical or cognitive limitations.

GOING FORWARD

The factors that influenced recent changes in long-term care settings are quite intermeshed. The culture change movement started in the 1980s and picked up significant momentum in the mid-1990s. About the same time, the National Endowment for the Arts and National Endowment for the Humanities sponsored a micro-conference on aging, which is said to mark the beginning of the dialogue on arts and aging. Simultaneously, the idea of active aging was emerging. The concept of active aging has been modified by aging-services providers to encompass holistic wellness for all people, not just younger elders living independently. Culture change, wellness, and the arts have all significantly influenced each other and the current landscape of activities in long-term care.

The United States is now in the midst of a huge demographic shift. In 2011, the first baby boomer turned sixty-five years old. While each generation of elders has brought new strengths, preferences, and expectations, the sheer number of those in the baby boom generation (those born between 1946 and 1964) will dramatically change the field of aging. Already, long-term care providers have noticed that younger elders often expect a higher level of involvement within the organization than previous generations. We can't predict exactly how the influx of baby boomers will influence the way activities are delivered in long-term care, but it's likely that boomers will continue to value health, physical activity, and personal gratification through vocation and independence.

As the field of aging continues to evolve, there's more work to be done. Most organizations acknowledge that culture change is an ongoing process. As new generations of elders and employees enter the world of long-term care, the culture of each organization must continue to evolve. Similarly, organizations are just embarking on the path of wellness. If holistic well-being is the goal, the entire organization must embrace every dimension. So, resident well-being can't be achieved if employee well-being isn't also achieved. And none of these things can happen in isolation. One or two staff people, or even a small team of staff people, can't be responsible for creating a culture of wellness and engagement — it must be in the DNA of the organization.

PENELOPE

I hope the Penelope Project sets the stage for more internal and external collaboration in long-term care. The most remarkable things that are happening in the aging-services field are not happening without the expertise, influence, and participation of the greater community. As aging-services providers invite artists, teachers, lawyers, computer programmers, gardeners, children, youth, and other elders into their communities, the experience of aging will improve for everyone.

As I meandered down the Luther Manor hallways, witnessing *Finding Penelope* as an audience member, I was filled with an overwhelming sense of hope. As organizations like Luther Manor, and those I've referenced above, continue to expand the definition of activities or life enrichment in long-term care, life in a nursing home will continue to improve for those who live and work there. Happily, it's clear to me that we are moving further and further away from my childhood experience of tap dancing my way through nursing homes.

WORKS CITED

Department of Health and Human Services (DHHS). 2006. CMS Manual System, Pub. 100-07 State Operations Provider Certification. https://www.cms.gov /Regulations-and-Guidance/Guidance/Transmittals/Downloads/R19SOMA .pdf (accessed October 9, 2015).

SOCIAL/CIVIC PRACTICE IN THE THEATRE
Michael Rohd

Currently, within institutional theatre organizations, community partnerships are most frequently developed to implement programming that surrounds the productions that appear on their main stage or stages. That programming exists to deepen the vision of the artists. Institutions sometimes retain partners beyond singular projects, returning to them for help on other projects when content seems aligned with the partner's constituency or mission. These partnerships are valuable; they can effectively build new relationships around meaningful, shared interests, and they help arts organizations broaden the scope of their presence in their local communities. But too commonly, they operate more like a monologue than a dialogue. The initiating impulse — the voice that puts out the call, so to speak — is the artist. The non-arts partner has a choice — the partner can listen, respond, or not. But rarely does the invitation to conversation, to co-creation, come from the partner.

In the current arts landscape, ideas of engagement, participation, and institution/audience relationship are seen as keys to both innovation and survival. There is a growing number of research studies and funding opportunities focused on audiences, community, and context — which is an indicator that energy is aligning for deep investigation and a commitment to advancement in these practices. The array of engagement approaches in professional theatre today takes many of its core impulses and tactics from the pioneering, community-based, often politically motivated artists of the 1960s and 1970s, through contemporary location-based ensembles and the most current branding, public relations, and interactivity/participation experts in the social media, business, and design sectors. The core impulses on this continuum are widely varied in underlying philosophy and goals. For us at Sojourn Theatre, the Penelope Project falls on a very specific point of a spectrum we use to consider cross-disciplinary engaged practice.

On this spectrum, performance that is considered to be *social practice* (a term that originally comes from the world of visual and installation art) initiates with artists' desire to explore/create a conceptual event or series of moments they design. The design and/or execution of the performance may engage non-artists in any number of ways: it may leverage non-arts partners and community resources; it may intend to specifically impact the social or civic life of the context in which it occurs in measurable ways; or it may intend to exist as an aesthetic interruption from which impact is to be derived in an open, interpretive manner. But alongside whatever social or civic needs the project addresses, the leading impulse and guiding energy is from the artist.

In performances that are considered to be *civic practice*, artists use the assets of their crafts in response to the goals of non-arts partners as discovered through ongoing dialogue. The impulse of what to make comes out of the relationship, not an artist-driven proposal. We find civic practice and social practice to be distinct modes of engaged activity, with civic practice aiming to help establish an area of artistic practice framed by intention and process. For much of Sojourn Theatre's fifteen years, we have made theatre work that functions more on the social practice continuum than the civic practice one. This is the case for Penelope. But, in the work of the project, in the learning we have experienced, in our relationship with Anne Basting, spots on the spectrum have blurred. They have overlapped and even reset. The prioritization of needs amidst an ever evolving partnership have led to a process where aspects of the work have clearly been determined by artist vision, but aspects have also clearly been guided by student, resident, and staff needs.

At Sojourn, we seek to name the assets that we bring to our partnerships. We seek invitations to new tables and to bring our assets with us. We try to listen and — when appropriate, when of use — offer our assets. We work to rethink the possibilities of partnership and create more opportunities to start with a partner's needs rather than our own programming.

We believe these goals help us increase our pool of stakeholders and redefine what participation in the arts means. We believe they increase meaningful opportunities for our artists to work in their communities and seed appreciation for creative public activity. We believe they increase desire for the assets that theatre artists bring to community settings beyond the traditional stage production — that more people will learn about the power of theatre by experiencing it through a variety of forms and encounters.

The Penelope Project is important for us as artists, as a company, and as citizens, because it has given us a unique opportunity to practice social, civic, and even studio practice as we worked with artists and non-artists alike to make a journey that we believe powerfully impacted quality of life for many involved. Ourselves included.

PENELOPE GOES TO COLLEGE . . . BUT DOES SHE GET ACCEPTED INTO THE THEATRE DEPARTMENT?
Jan Cohen-Cruz

Where does Penelope fit in the higher education landscape? How is an inter-disciplinary, on- and off-campus, multiyear project with a core nonuniversity partner justified as an appropriate component of the college experience so as to gain a foothold in the institution as a whole? What of the relationship between such a project and its disciplinary base? Specifically, how do cross-sector performance initiatives that don't align with strictly aesthetic criteria secure a place at the table of a theatre department? Or do art world parame-ters require trained actors and content that can be *about* a social issue but not contribute to *improving* it? In what follows, I share some thoughts, first, on how community-engaged learning/art like the Penelope Project becomes part of the culture of higher education and, second, on how it establishes a home in its artistic discipline.

Validating publically engaged projects like Penelope within higher educa-tion is often grounded in the "serving the public good" aspect of most univer-sities' missions. This value is reflected in the propagation of "service learning" on campuses. However, I am among those who prefer to frame initiatives like the Penelope Project as public scholarship, which both more accurately de-scribes them than does service and gets closer to the heart of higher educa-tion's purpose. Thus a more useful philosophical container is civic profession-alism, which proposes that a higher education provide students with (1) the capacity to think critically, (2) a pathway to a career, and (3) the experience of applying their discipline in the world as part of being a citizen. Scott J. Peters (codirector of the consortium Imagining America: Artists and Schol-ars in Public Life) notes that civic professionalism "casts professionals' iden-tities, roles, and expertise around a civic mission. It places scholars inside public life, rather than apart from or above it, working alongside their fellow citizens on questions and issues of public importance" (2003). Civic profes-sionalism is a bridge between intellectual and practical learning, and between vocational goals and the common good. It responds to student yearning to do something meaningful. It aligns pedagogy with both preparation for a career and a discipline-based experience of active citizenship, at the same time preserving the breadth and nuance of inquiry that are hallmarks of the arts and humanities.

As pedagogy, the Penelope Project was fertile ground for students to develop critical thinking and learning-by-doing, collaborating on a theatre piece with elders at Luther Manor. It was what Ernest Boyer calls the scholarship of application (1990), providing a context for students to use what they'd learned about devising: creating/improvising original theatre in a real situation. More, students were face-to-face with older people who brought the subject matter alive. Evaluators noted this comment by one student as typical of other student participants: "It is amazing being around these women . . . an enlightening experience. At first I was terrified. Now, it's funny to think I was. I want to do this again. Are there other courses like this?" (Penelope Project Program Evaluation 2013, 67). The learning could not have stretched the students as profoundly had it stayed entirely in a classroom with participants all within a few years of each other in age.

As for career path, being part of Penelope's development opened the students to collaborative ways of making theatre and expanded their horizons regarding with whom, where, and about what one can do so. This knowledge was enhanced by the range of their activities — as workshop facilitators and theatre makers — and of the participants: University of Wisconsin-Milwaukee faculty and students from different departments (especially theatre and gerontology), Sojourn Theatre members, and residents and staff of the senior facility.

As a conduit to civic participation, Penelope provided the experience of how meaningful theatre can be when concretely embedded in the world. Penelope enhanced the lives of several hundred people — the students, senior residents and staff, and audiences. All who participated were part of an enacted civic dialogue about the joys and vicissitudes of aging.

But cross-sector (for example, from the sectors of the arts and long-term care) and community-based learning are often hard to justify within a discipline. Making a case for Penelope in a theatre department depends partly on both the tenacity and the artistic credentials of the instigator (Basting in this case), the perspectives of the actual people in powerful positions, and how scholars in that field see engaged, interdisciplinary work. I turn now to this factor.

Shannon Jackson, the director of the Arts Research Center at UC Berkeley, has looked at contemporary visual and performing arts engaged in what the visual art world calls social practice. While not the only scholar to do so, she importantly bridges the art world — with her deep knowledge of the history of the avant-garde and her theoretical acumen — and the potential value of social institutions, as most fully manifested in her publication about Chicago's Hull House settlement, *Lines of Activity* (2000). She can thus question "models of political engagement that measure artistic radicality by its degree of anti-institutionality," placing equal importance on "art forms that help us imagine sustainable social institutions" (Jackson 2011, 14). She and other insightful, articulate scholars and practitioners play a crucial role in validating artistic initiatives that cross into social territory. They offer an alternative perspective to traditional scholars for whom such projects can seem to be "theater-lite, distracting students from the 'real' pursuit of their craft" (Basting 2013).

Given higher education itself as a culture, it is significant that artists/scholars at other colleges and universities, most of whom who have been at their institutions for a relatively long time, are also integrating cross-sector campus and community performance projects. Cindy Cohen is developing an arts and social justice focus at Brandeis; Buzz Alexander has long provided an opportunity to be involved in the arts in the criminal justice system through the University of Michigan. Michael Rohd initiated *How to End Poverty* — a combination play, lecture, interactive workshop, and public conversation — as part of Northwestern University's main stage season. At Virginia Tech, longtime theatre professor Bob Leonard initiated the Directing and Public Dialogue program through which students collaborate with local artists and community-based organizations around sensitive issues.

In 2011, for example, Leonard worked closely with student John Catherwood-Ginn to initiate the Building Home project with students, local artists, and other Virginia Tech theatre faculty, in partnership with the southwest Virginia regional planning office. The planning office wanted to increase public involvement and input about the future of the New River Valley, which they knew meant going beyond the surveys and public hearings on which they typically relied. Building Home was created to use storytelling and theatre-making techniques to facilitate and stimulate such public conversation, especially among people who did not usually participate in civic efforts.

Graduates of initiatives like Penelope — often called applied theatre — who go on to make meaningful careers are another measure of such projects' value. In 2014, I brought in two former students from my own years of teaching at NYU to facilitate sessions of my History of Community-Based Theatre class.

One, Matt Sergi, is now a professor of Medieval Studies (and has written eloquently about the ties between community-based and medieval theatre); the other, Monica Hunken, is a performance activist who has done powerful work with Occupy Wall Street as well as Reverend Billy and his Church of Stop Shopping, among others. Former student Jamie Haft now works with Roadside Theater in Appalachia; Kiyoko McCrae now works with Junebug Productions in New Orleans; and both Haft and Kevin Bott are on staff at Imagining America, in Syracuse. Bott, Imaging America's associate director, has also created a community-based theatre in Syracuse called Dream Freedom Revival. Michael Rohd was a student of Bob Leonard's and, besides starting Sojourn Theatre in the years since, served as an advisor on his Building Home project.

Projects like Penelope do encounter challenges. Basting acknowledged that sometimes community members are skeptical of higher education. The fear is that academics are only focused on their research goals and not on community benefit. Within the university, competition for resources is a challenge, be it among faculty for students in their classes and projects, staff-time for the additional labor of projects over classes, and indirect funds from grants that often must be managed by the lead investigator's department. Department heads may not recognize how much release time a faculty investigator needs to carry out such projects or how to translate such initiatives in terms of expectations for promotion.

Nonetheless, Basting noted that the benefits of higher education as a platform far outweigh the challenges. Basting avowed that the Penelope Project could not have happened at that level of professionalism and knowledge-generation without the multilayered support provided by a university, with contributions from faculty of several disciplines (especially technical theatre and gerontology), staff, and students; a professional theatre company; and Luther Manor's staff and residents. She has found that the increasing focus among funders on outcomes makes it necessary to wrap smart and significant evaluation around work of this kind. Higher education can support such evaluation with its institutional review board structures and collaborative partners across social science and clinical disciplines. Trans-disciplinary collaborations such as Penelope add gravitas because of the additional expertise involved and the clear engagement of disciplines and sectors beyond traditional theatre. Basting summarized: "Higher education for me has been a very strong base that enabled us to receive more funding, forge trans-disciplinary partnerships, and coordinate complex community partnerships with the re-sources at hand" (Basting 2013).

To make higher education a more congenial, supportive context from which to collaborate across disciplines and sectors, Basting calls for conver-sations about how the infrastructures are different for different disciplines:

> We can't truly grow trans-disciplinary work until we have a basic understanding of how our fields operate. What are the products of your research? What is innovation? How is your work measured/valued within the institution? What is your teaching load and why? What do you need to get promoted? What makes you vulnerable? (Basting 2013)

She recognizes both such exchanges internal to the academy—between, say, professors of theatre and social work or nursing—and related questions across the sectors of higher education and community-based organizations as in her partnerships with Luther Manor staff. Such conversations are equally necessary within the discourse of higher education's purpose and regarding performance as a discipline, so that initiatives like Penelope can find a home in colleges and universities and art departments, at the same time helping ex-pand our very understanding of what performance does in the world.

WORKS CITED

Basting, A. 2013. Interview with the author via email, March 15.

Boyer, E. 1990. *Scholarship Reconsidered: Priorities of the Professoriate*. Menlo Park, CA: Carnegie Foundation for the Advancement of Teaching.

Jackson, S. 2000. *Lines of Activity: Performance, Historiography, Hull-House Domesticity*. Ann Arbor: University of Michigan Press.

Jackson, S. 2011. *Social Works: Performing Art, Supporting Publics*. New York and London: Routledge.

Penelope Project Program Evaluation. 2013. www.thepenelopeproject.com/links /materials (accessed March 16, 2015).

Peters, S. 2003. "Reconstructing Civic Professionalism in Academic Life: A Response to Mark Wood's Paper, 'From Service to Solidarity.'" *Journal of Higher Education Outreach and Engagement* 8 (2): 183–98.

PART TWO: *Building Partnerships and Charting a Path*

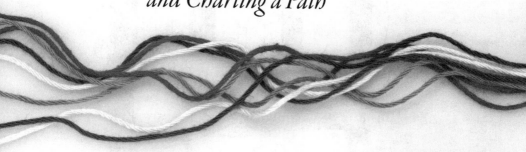

Penelope is the discovery of something spectacular while patiently waiting. It is shared courage, shared story, and shared journey.
—*Nikki Zaleski, Sojourn Performer*

This section examines how the partnerships formed and how we took our first steps in developing Penelope. In a lively dialogue, Anne Basting (University of Wisconsin–Milwaukee [UWM]) and Beth Meyer-Arnold (Luther Manor) tease out their memories of the original impulses for the project and how the partnerships helped create its own structure. As always, the story exists somewhere between a variety of memories and points of view. Similarly, Basting and Michael Rohd (Sojourn) share memories of how the collaboration with Sojourn began and how the project was structured to facilitate a deep and extensive participation from professional theatre artists. In a shared essay, Basting and UWM Department of Theatre colleague Robin Mello describe how the project was structured to engage undergraduate students and to meet their unique, semester-based curricular needs. To complete our focus on first steps, Anne Basting charts the evolution of the project's funding and evaluation plans, and Basting and Mello look at the unique power of myth for the Penelope Project and its power as an underlying framework.

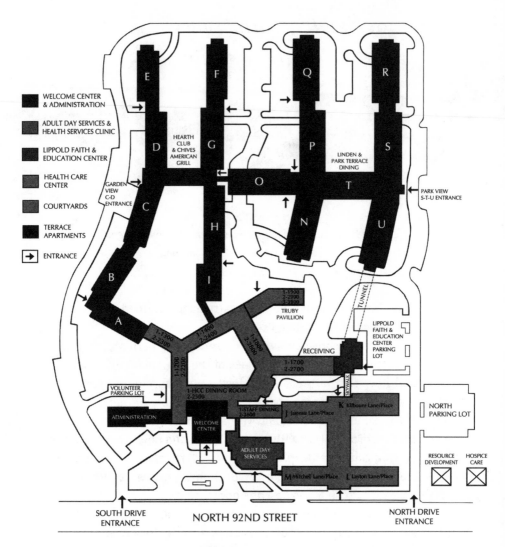

WELCOME CENTER & ADMINISTRATION

ADULT DAY SERVICES & HEALTH SERVICES CLINIC

LIPPOLD FAITH & EDUCATION CENTER

HEALTH CARE CENTER

COURTYARDS

TERRACE APARTMENTS

ENTRANCE

E
F
Q
R
D
G
P
S
HEARTH CLUB & CHIVES AMERICAN GRILL
LINDEN & PARK TERRACE DINING
GARDEN VIEW C-D ENTRANCE
O
PARK VIEW S-T-U ENTRANCE
C
H
N
T
B
I
U
A

1-1900
2-2900
3-3900
TRUBY PAVILLION

TUNNEL

1-1300
2-2300
1-1400
2-2400
1-1600
2-2600
LIPPOLD FAITH & EDUCATION CENTER PARKING LOT

RECEIVING

1-1200
2-2200
1-1700
2-2700

SKYWALK

VOLUNTEER PARKING LOT

1-HCC DINING ROOM
2-2500

1-STAFF DINING
2-2600

J Juneau Lane/Place
K Kilbourn Lane/Place

NORTH PARKING LOT

ADMINISTRATION

WELCOME CENTER

ADULT DAY SERVICES

M Mitchell Lane/Place
L Layton Lane/Place

RESOURCE DEVELOPMENT
HOSPICE CARE

SOUTH DRIVE ENTRANCE

NORTH 92ND STREET

NORTH DRIVE ENTRANCE

North

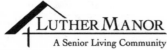

LUTHER MANOR
A Senior Living Community

4545 N. 92nd Street • Wauwatosa, WI 53225
(414) 464-3880 • FAX (414) 464-9050 • www.luthermanor.org

MISC20120618-07

WHAT IS LUTHER MANOR?

Anne Basting

Luther Manor is a retirement community that provides a continuum of care—from independent apartments (the Terrace) to assisted living (the Courtyards), skilled nursing (the Health Care Center), and day services for older adults living at home (the Day Center). The community is managed by the United Lutheran Program for Aging, a nonprofit of more than seventy affiliated congregations. Luther Manor opened its doors to its first twelve residents in 1961 and has grown to become a small village—covering over a million square feet. Over seven hundred people live at Luther Manor, and over seven hundred people work there on various shifts throughout the week. It sits nestled on twenty-nine acres next to a golf course in Wauwatosa, a first-ring suburb of Milwaukee. When Penelope began in 2009, Luther Manor's Day Center had a long history of collaborating with UWM faculty and students. Basting had pioneered the TimeSlips project there in 1998, and UWM professor Gerald Weisman and former student Lyn Geboy worked closely with director of the Day Center Beth Meyer-Arnold on establishing a "person-centered" (rather than staff-centered) approach to both programming and architectural design.

EVOLUTION OF AN IDEA: IN DIALOGUE
Anne Basting and Beth Meyer-Arnold

Basting (UWM) and Meyer-Arnold (Luther Manor) had known each other and worked together on various projects for fifteen years before Basting proposed the idea for the Penelope Project. Luther Manor was one of the four original pilot sites for the development of TimeSlips, an improvisational storytelling technique used with people with cognitive disabilities that Basting began in 1998. Meyer-Arnold was a member of the leadership council for the Center on Age & Community that Basting directed from 2003 to 2013.

Anne: It was a handful of years ago now — the origins are blurry to me. Do you remember how this whole thing started?

Beth: I remember that you came and started talking about doing some kind of project that would engage the residents in thinking about issues of home — what is home, leaving home — and loneliness, leaving, and waiting. You thought those were big issues for older people and especially people living in care settings. And then you mentioned the *Odyssey* and specifically the story of Penelope. That was what I remember as a first conversation. And of course I had no idea how we were going to get residents and students on the same page about something like that. But I knew that projects with you always turn out wonderful and that we would figure it out.

Also, in those first conversations we were thinking about doing this in the nursing home — that those were nursing homes issues. Especially waiting. When you talked about the number of students (twenty to thirty), I said that we needed to open this up to all the units. And then of course we saw that those were issues for everyone, everywhere. And then the adventure/romance from the story of Penelope really took over and intrigued everyone. It wasn't the issues that drew them, but how exciting and interesting this could be for everyone. That changed quickly what this project could be about.

Anne: What were you thinking might come out of it at the beginning?

Beth: I knew that there would be some kind of "give-back" production with the students. Maybe a one-act play or a scene that they would write using the older adults' words. And then when I met the theatre company, I really thought it was going to be a stage play. Three acts. Everyone watching the play together. I really had no concept what it was going to be like — that it would really involve the way that people were living in the Courtyards and nursing home. That it would show a little slice of what life was like here. Sometimes I think it was kind of like this musical inside somebody's home. When you think about the fact that we moved the actual play from the Welcome Center to the dining room and to the nurse's station and social worker's office — I really had no idea that was possible from a theatre production standpoint. I never wondered if it was going to be possible from a care center perspective. We just kept going and begging forgiveness from people. There were a few sort of tiny little voices saying, "That's too much!" But you were really good at having the meetings and asking people, "How can we work around that?"

Anne: In my work with TimeSlips [see www.timeslips.org], we created improvised, original stories in care settings and then produced the plays inspired by those stories in professional settings. I wanted to bring those two elements together — to create the materials and stage the production in the same place and bring in an outside audience. In the earlier TimeSlips play productions, we were asking audiences to think about people with memory loss as being capable of creativity and meaningful expression. In the last TimeSlips play in New York, we had professional actors playing people with memory loss. But now I wanted to have them play themselves. Could we do it? How? What would the audience's experience be like to be in the "home" as a performance space?

Beth: And we were saying, can we push this a little bit further? And if we do, what will happen? What will be the benefits? The barriers? The problems? Where will people say, "That's too far. That's too much?" There was a little bit of that — there was. There were some people who never understood what we were doing and who felt that it was an interruption of people's lives and the work we need to get done. But those were few and far between. Now I realize there will always be those people — and that you can't let those people stop the efforts to improve the culture of care.

Anne: I also remember that you had done such incredible work with person-centered care in the Adult Day Center at Luther Manor and were eager to spread it throughout the whole care campus at Luther Manor, but it had been difficult for it to get traction.

Beth: People say, "Well, it works there in adult day, but it'll never work here." Really, I don't think people on staff here even knew what "it" was.

Anne: I think part of your interest was in seeing if this might jump-start that process a bit. The person-centered roots of this kind of approach — inviting input from residents; echoing, affirming, and shaping their responses; and supporting creative expression and turning it into art — could create an experiential model for the programming staff on other units.

Pretty quickly we realized that we were up to something quite radical — we were embedding improvisation and collaboration into a whole care center — a whole, hyper-regulated system that is designed to *reduce* and manage risk, not open to it. We were asking them to open themselves to the unknown and create it together.

Beth: What if the way we care for older adults REALLY was about the people who live here, their words, how they spend their days? What if it was about doing what *they* want to do? When you realize how mind-numbing these care systems can be — especially in a nursing home — where people don't have their own spaces to go back to, or staff think people can't be in their own private space. It's so hard for a lot of staff to imagine what real "engagement" can really be. We [the staff] go back to things that are rote for us. Or we think, "Old people like this." Or this "one person likes it," therefore all older people will like it. It's also so risky — to try something new feels risky for staff and administration. People feel more comfortable doing things they know how to do, like play bingo and ask trivia questions.

EVOLUTION OF AN IDEA: IN DIALOGUE
Anne Basting and Michael Rohd

Basting and Rohd had known each other from the early days of graduate school but never collaborated on a project before. With Rohd's serendipitous move to the Midwest and some good timing, the two realized they had found their first opportunity to collaborate.

Anne: In my memory, I was happy to see that you had landed at Northwestern, just ninety minutes down the road from me. I was looking forward to touching base again after many years. We had started out in the Theatre and Social Change group at ATHE [Association for Theatre in Higher Education] as graduate students at the same time, and our work had grown and evolved in some interesting ways over years. We even both collaborated with renowned theatre artist Ping Chong, but at separate times. I had gone deeply into the field of aging and the arts, but was feeling a little distant from the arts part after eight years in administration. I was looking for a way back, and had an idea for a big project percolating in my mind. It seemed a perfect moment, if a bit overdue, to reconnect. So we met for coffee in Evanston . . .

Michael: I was really intrigued with the work you had been doing in aging and the arts. It seemed that my growing interest in cross-sector work [arts-based practice that engaged with partners in non-arts centered fields] could really be enhanced by learning more about what you do, and potentially by working together on something. I was looking to develop more Sojourn work in the Midwest at this time too. Sojourn was busy on the West Coast and on the East Coast, but not anywhere near Chicago, where I actually was now living. So, we met for coffee in Evanston . . .

Anne: "Are you working on anything now?" you asked. I remember saying, "I have an idea, but it's tricky because I don't have my own theatre company in Milwaukee, and there really isn't a deep tradition of deeply community-engaged, site-specific theatre that is taken seriously as art."

Of course you asked me what it was—and asked all the right questions to help me tease out the idea. That idea revolved around telling the *Odyssey* from Penelope's point of view and her twenty years of waiting, as devised from engaging with residents of a nursing home, who are similarly assumed to be sitting around, waiting. We would aim to get an audience to understand that care facilities can be so much more than waiting rooms.

I wasn't pitching you the project. But in the middle of my description, and your astute questions, I think we both realized that this was indeed the project for our first collaboration together. "I think I know the perfect director," you said. "Can she come to a think tank in two weeks about how to radically transform activities in long-term care?" I asked. And she did.

Michael: Maureen Towey entered the picture. She's an artist that came to Sojourn through a Princess Grace fellowship in 2006 that allowed her to spend a good part of 2007 in Portland with us (when we were still based there). She is an excellent director, but also a really creative thinker and an innovator. She works some in the rock-and-roll and concert world; she has worked in the community-development world. She has passionate interests outside theatre, yet she also strongly identifies as a maker of new performance. She had become, by the time you and I had coffee in Evanston, a trusted colleague and friend, and clearly an artist to bring into the conversation you and I were beginning.

Anne: Once Maureen entered the picture, she really became the core link to Sojourn. You were there in key phone meetings, and you came up to Milwaukee at key times to provide really valuable feedback on where we were and particularly on how we were conceptualizing things. The project really was perfect for Sojourn — but I was also very struck by how this project was a unique challenge for Sojourn too. This was the first time that Sojourn would be doing a site-specific work at a place where people were living. As a space, Luther Manor had more than symbolic meaning. Seven hundred people live at Luther Manor, and seven hundred people work there. It is a space with deeply entrenched daily rhythms. Every step we took there was in collaboration with staff and residents. This meant that collaboration couldn't be shallow — it was in every breath, smile, and eye contact. It was everything.

SHAPING THE PROJECT STRUCTURE FROM
A CARE PERSPECTIVE: IN DIALOGUE
Anne Basting and Beth Meyer-Arnold

Anne: As we designed the project, were there issues that you remember being a challenge? What things felt important to put in place?

Beth: In the beginning, I was thinking in a very "long-term care continuum framework" for how logistically this project would work. How could we hear all the voices of all the different people at Luther Manor? We would want a group to talk to those people who were living in the community and coming here [Day Center] for services; people in residential assisted living; people living in our independent apartments; and people receiving skilled nursing services. That is the current way that a lot of CCRCs [Continuing Care Retirement Communities] are organized. I thought this would be a great way to hear the voices of *all* the people who live or receive services here. These four areas had never before collaborated on a project or programming together.

At the beginning, I wasn't thinking of all the other people at Luther Manor. But as we got going and people got really interested in what was happening — I think we realized that there were other voices. You were very aware of that before I was. It's interesting the way you were aware of the voice of Julianne [the receptionist] — "Luther Manor, how may I direct your call?" That ritual sort of way that we all started to notice things differently — through you noticing Julianne and how she was really starting to interact with the students and theatre folks.

We thought we should have four groups of students facilitating discussions — one in each of the four care areas. Then we asked, who are the key people in those groups? I do remember that the people I thought were key at the beginning weren't ultimately the ones that proved the most helpful. I had a conversation with David Keller [CEO], and he recommended that we connect with the case managers. I had been focusing on the activity directors. But when we got connected to the case managers, things really clicked. These are social workers who really know the residents very well.

I also remember that the first time we met with an administration group—how important it was for them to hear about the project from you. The university and theatre people—you were using theatre language—it was so different from our language—it really got their attention. And David [Keller] knew that you and I had had other successful partnerships/collaborations—with you and with students. That was really important. Having you come early enough and talk about this in a language that was different than our medical language, that was very important.

Anne: Why was that important?

Beth: The expert is always twenty-five miles away. An outsider's perspective could help raise their interest that this would be different than the run of the mill "entertainment model" project where musicians or artists come in and residents enjoy and applaud their efforts. I think you were able to say, "We are thinking about doing something different." I've been saying it—but they heard it from you using different language. People began saying, "Yeah, I think this is going to be different." I remember you said the next thing we need to find out is how the life of Luther Manor works. Like when/where does the laundry go? The ambulance? The meals? The medication? Etc. And people were like—wow! They really want to know what the real, everyday life of Luther Manor is like. How do things get announced on the public announcement system? I remember looking around at the faces of the people and when you were starting to ask those questions—that was really important.

Anne: I remember asking, "As part of the performance, is there any place we can't go?" I remember David [Keller] saying, "I don't think there's anywhere that is off-limits." And I thought, we've crossed a threshold just now.

Beth: We found out we couldn't go out the window—

Anne: But we could! We did!

Beth: The maintenance team thought we couldn't. When they saw the performers doing it in rehearsal they called the CEO. But then David [Keller] asked, "Is this necessary to the plot of the play? Yes? Then go ahead."

Anne: I remember that day-long training workshop in April of the year before [2010]. We held it in the Adult Day Center on a Saturday. It was an important first step in learning from each other.

Beth: Now, looking back, I would have invited different people to that initial training session. I think we had some of the right people there—but if I was giving advice to people now, I would invite as many people as you possibly can. Wouldn't it have been cool to have had someone from switchboard, receptionist, dietary, security — or maintenance? And more CNAs [certified nursing assistants]. I was thinking of it very much from the activities programming perspective, and included some of the nursing personnel as well. We didn't have that buy-in from the health care folks, nursing or CNAs, that we had hoped. We got interest from people we never thought we would — but looking back now, I would have included a wider variety of people in that early training. And maybe it didn't need to be a whole day — maybe just two hours, and in shifts to reach more people.

Anne: It was very effective for the programming folks — I hadn't anticipated that they would go ahead and start programming activities inspired by the Penelope story so quickly. When we had a check-in phone call in September and they started telling us about all the programming they were doing, I thought, "Wait! You have to talk to us about what you're doing!" Especially Jeanne [Life Enrichment staff person in the Health Care Center], who was just picking it up and running with it.

Beth: And there was a lot of the behind the scenes during that time with Ellie Rose [visual artist and person-centered care specialist in the Day Center]. She saw it as an opportunity to connect with the other programming areas. She was thinking, "Why aren't we inviting people from other areas to share programming?" That was a really great vehicle for her to start connecting with other activity programmers and join efforts.

Anne: Are there any other structural elements that seemed really crucial?

Beth: Looking back — you can never tell the families enough about it. Those families that got involved, the daughters were such dedicated fans — they really got the value of it. If we could have gotten more families involved earlier and understood the power of this for families — as a time for people to visit — we didn't fully appreciate how powerful that was. We could have used that more for everything. From the Luther Manor side — the public relations, the feelings of well-being between families who have to have their loved one in an institution who are proud of what we are doing. The university outreach — including those people earlier on — to talk about it, to raise awareness in the bigger world. I know you were worried about how you would handle a bigger audience. But there were two pastors and their wives who were so engaged with this — they were hearing about it for two years. They were part of our home/community-based services and were hearing about it from me every meeting. This was really interesting to them. They were there with their wives. One was at the premiere of the documentary at UWM. We sat together to watch it. That was also something that we didn't realize how powerful that could have been — to connect other audiences or publics.

Anne: Structurally, I was really moved by the final focus group that we held to review what happened. It felt really important to have that group expanded from just programming staff to include administrators, family, residents, staff from all over.

Beth: From my standpoint, other administrators didn't ever completely understand why it was important to get input from other staff. People could understand why it was important to get my input, input from activity people, and the residents — but other people never really understood why it was important to get Julianne's [switchboard operator] feedback. Or feedback from people in other departments. I could have done a better job helping them understand that. Even nursing leaders. The nursing people were always invited. And the administrators. But I don't know that they ever really understood why it would have been important to have CNAs involved and giving input on and framing this project. I think that these projects are still seen as "activities." Maybe as you talk about it — maybe it's the project. Maybe it is that language. Maybe there is a different word — words — that would be more in the language of medical people. I don't know. They are pretty entrenched in their language. There are some nursing leaders who have a different language. They get that it can affect the life of the community in such a positive way — so the more people involved in it, the better.

Anne: What about the idea that we gave the whole project some real time to develop?

Beth: Yes. And I think the student semester-and-year schedule is a good one. It's a comfortable framework. People know that schedule — they've known it since they've started going to school. So that feels good and gave us that external timeline — so you didn't feel like you were making up something with no direction. I loved it too that the theatre people were here for a week or ten days at a time — that was a luxury. So even if they are working with a local group, having them be there day after day for a week or two, a couple different times — that would be very nice. That was such a sign of something new and different.

Anne: It was an infusion.

Beth: It was also the way that you had the theatre crew eating lunch with residents in the staff dining room — all that was great strategy.

SHAPING THE PROJECT STRUCTURE FROM
AN ARTS PERSPECTIVE: IN DIALOGUE
Anne Basting and Michael Rohd

Anne: One of the first things we had to do was figure out how to structure the project — the stages, the duration, the goals, the objectives, the outcomes. This meant figuring out when [and for how long] to bring in the Sojourn artists. Together we created multiple phases and decided to bring Sojourn members in for residencies during each phase, with consistent phone and electronic communication in between. Here is that basic structure:

APRIL 2009–AUGUST 2010
Partnership Development: Sojourn's Maureen Towey came to Milwaukee to participate in a think tank called "Radically Transforming Activities in Long-Term Care."
Michael Rohd and Towey were in residence in April 2010 for a cross-partner training workshop at Luther Manor and a presentation on the project at the National Association of Activity Professionals annual conference held in Milwaukee.

SEPTEMBER 2010–DECEMBER 2010
Creative Research: Sojourn's Shannon Scrofano (Designer), Rebecca Martinez (Performer), James Hart (Performer), Towey (Director), and Rohd were *in residence for one week* in October 2010.

JANUARY 2011–MARCH 2011
Devising and Performance: Sojourn's Scrofano, Hart, Martinez, Towey, and two additional performers (Nikki Zaleski and Daniel Cohen) are in residence for *one week of devising* in January 2011. They return for *four weeks of rehearsal and performance* from mid-February through mid-March.

APRIL 2011–ONGOING
Disseminating: Sojourn's Rohd, Scrofano, and Towey return for a retreat in Milwaukee in July 2012 to craft an outline and approach to writing a book. A documentary, website, and educational guide are completed.

Anne: How did you arrive at this structure for this project? What's important when you're sitting down to come up with a structure like this?

Michael: For any project that Sojourn goes through, we're always trying to find the right way of working for the specific project. It's not like there's a formula—but there is a progression of steps that are common to any devised project, whether it's community engaged or studio based. I certainly think we went through it on this project. Those steps are:

(1) Starting Impulse;
(2) Research/Partner-Building;
(3) Generative Process;
(4) Authorship Construction;
(5) Rehearse/Refine;
(6) Production Event;
(7) Resulting Ongoing Process.

Of course, those phases aren't discrete; sometimes they bleed and blur and jump back and forth, but you have to go through all those phases. I would certainly say we went through that kind of progression in a way that was unique to this project.

Anne: Did you see this project as being especially different or challenging, or was the structure simply what you were used to?

Michael: I think the meta- or macro-structure was familiar, but there were really unique challenges. One of them was that we were making work in a place where people live. Not just about people's lives, but actually in a facility where living occurs. All the issues of research, partner-building, generation, and authorship were constantly in dialogue with notions of home and daily activity. The revelation that seemed most important early on—which was really yours—was that the dramaturgy [story/plot] of the facility had to become a skeleton for the theatrical event. We had to embed the way the place functioned into the way the play moved. That was an exciting evolution in thinking about site-based work, participatory work, and devised work. The dramaturgy was very real and daily, and many people's lives were attached to it in concrete ways. Trying to make the piece of theatre live on that dramaturgy made for a better chance of success in the partnerships; it also made for a more exciting theatricality for people to experience, because it was so organically connected to the bones of the place we were in. This is something I've taken on in conversations about civic partnerships now: this notion that systems have their own dramaturgy, and you can think about intervening, or you can think about embedding, or blending around, or working within. All too often, in the arts, we think about whatever system we're landing in as the thing we have to negotiate in order to do the thing we really want to do. This really makes a good case for the fact that the most meaningful work will take place when you learn the system. That's not to say you can't confront it, challenge it, subvert it, whisper to it, and all those things — but you do have to find a way to work with the system, dramaturgically.

Anne: And changes to the system happen just through your presence in that system, by the way that you work with your own integrity. We saw that happen with Penelope pretty clearly. In some ways you're making change simply by being part of the system, listening to it, and echoing it back, so that its members see it and recognize changes they want to make themselves.

Michael: We've made shows with students in university settings before. But in this case there was a lot of different interaction going on between the project and the school, the students, and the facility. How does that fit in for you, structurally? Was it a necessity? What do you feel the student involvement contributed to Penelope, other than resources, that could not have been accomplished without that partnership?

Anne: Working with the students, I was considering three things. First, I was thinking about how students in general could be involved in the long term. Hopefully, we could continue this work where we're doing embedded, engaged learning through the arts, and trying to make that part of the curriculum in an ongoing way. Second, I knew from collaborating with care facilities before that there is a power in an ongoing presence of the next generation. There's an opening that happens through the energy that younger people bring, and through the opportunity for residents to engage with that generation. Finally, because the collaborating theatre company was not Milwaukee-based, having students involved gave us an opportunity to be on the ground every single week with that energy and presence. That was really helpful. As an educator, it's just such powerful work for the students to be involved in, and I wanted to make sure it happened — but importantly, in terms of my own time, entwining my research and creative practice with my teaching was very practical for me as an artist.

Was this process unique or difficult because Sojourn wasn't in residence in the location where the work was taking place? The communication systems feel very important to set up, and that feels like part of the structure that isn't addressed in the progressive steps you mentioned before. How crucial is that kind of communication, in your eyes?

Michael: I think there are two factors. Sometimes there are partnerships that you have more contact with than the other leaders in the artistic team. In that case, it's important for those conversations to be ongoing, so it doesn't jump ahead without the engagement of the whole artistic team in all those moments of decision-making, which are constantly happening, even when we don't notice it. We need to make certain that we are in conversation through that process, or they'll go three steps forward in a creative model and we will have missed a chance to have input at a significant moment.

Anne: I agree. Whoever the team is on the ground, whether they're students or not, they're making creative discoveries constantly. With the Luther Manor staff there was this moment where we realized that they were already embedding the project in their daily activities. There was creative advancement happening with the staff and the residents that we didn't even know about, even though we were on the ground. Keeping that conversation going felt crucial, not just to keep Sojourn linked in, but to keep the faculty and students woven in to what the staff and residents were doing. We always had to make sure we were aware of what leaps were happening.

Michael: In addition to knowing what leaps are happening, there's this tension in doing any kind of community-engaged project, whether it's social practice or civic practice: What role does the artist's expertise and virtuosity have when one starts making decisions about authorship? We could make fifteen shows with undergrads that are consensus driven, and they wouldn't be satisfying to us as artists, because they hadn't gone through rigorous honing in collaboration with the more experienced artists. There's keeping tabs, and there's also knowing at what moment is it necessary that the artistic team have moments of leadership and filtering. Ongoing conversation is important for any project, but both because of the duration of these projects, the number of people involved, and the heavy amount of work you've been moving forward, it was especially important in Penelope.

Anne: Is there anything about the structure of the project that you wish we could have done differently? What would you have added if you had fantasy amounts of funding?

Michael: I wouldn't have changed much. With fantasy amounts of funding, I would have Rebecca and James [Sojourn performers] more able to spend time in residence on the ground with you and the team. We did well; they got there frequently. But I think every time Maureen [Towey, the director] and I were there, I would have them in just because they would bring different voices and perspective from which we would benefit as an ensemble. In fantasy funding world, I would have a few more of the collaborators present more often.

SHAPING THE PROJECT STRUCTURE FROM A TEACHING/LEARNING PERSPECTIVE

Robin Mello and Anne Basting

We are both scholars and artists in a theatre department in the only stand-alone school of the arts in the University of Wisconsin System (twenty-six campuses). At the University of Wisconsin–Milwaukee, our department began as a professional theatre company with a master's in fine arts, with a solid focus on training theatre professionals. Over the years, it has maintained its focus on learning through production but shifted toward an undergraduate program. UWM is an urban, public university with a high percentage of first-generation students. Our students commonly work two or three jobs to meet the costs of their education.

When we began conceptualizing the Penelope Project from the perspective of educators, the question facing us was clear. How could we embed a multiyear project like Penelope into the undergraduate curriculum in a way that would serve both students' curricular needs (courses they need toward their degree) and the goals/framework of the larger project? To get through a degree program in four to five years, students need flexibility to come in and out of a project through different classes that would fulfill their various requirements. Being engaged in a project through all three or four semesters would not be possible for the vast majority of students. Before the project began in earnest, we sat down together at a whiteboard and outlined a multiyear structure that would fit within our department of theatre's focus on production; our students' need for flexibility; and the project's need for consistent and deep presence of students and their creative energy.

Our first step was to create a one-semester, undergraduate research project to help fuel the research and development phase of the project. In fall 2009, we put out a call for research assistants: undergraduate students interested in participating in a dramaturgical seminar that would hone students' skills in theatrical research and provide background materials for Penelope programs and activities. The UWM Office of Undergraduate Research's SURF program (Support for Undergraduate Research Fellows) granted six students an opportunity to engage in this work.

The SURF undergraduate research project, entitled *Penelope Project Re-*

search Team, was implemented as a group dramaturgical research study with eighteen weeks of seminar meetings. The students' goal would be to create an educational guide that would serve to welcome people to the Penelope Project, from residents and staff to artists and future students. We tracked and compiled all information and research activities using the Desire-to-Learn (D2L) online course site. D2L is similar to a shared files/blog/website for each UWM course. Much of this material was subsequently used as foundational texts for fall 2010 course development and as groundwork for creating the play *Finding Penelope* as well.

Our second step was to plan our teaching and creative workload for the following year. Anne already was the faculty of record for Playwriting, while Robin was the instructor of Storytelling. We decided that Playwriting would focus on engaging students in the Sojourn Theatre devising model of play creation, while Storytelling would provide students with opportunities to learn and engage with the ancient myth of Odysseus and Penelope as well as explore intergenerational, ethnographic storytelling (gathering stories from listening to and interviewing people). This overlapping two-course curriculum was based on several past course projects (460 TimeSlips Creative Storytelling,[1] 460 Elder Tales,[2] and 460 Milwaukee Stories[3]), which had served as pilots for student engagement at Luther Manor. Because the project demanded collaboration among these students, we decided to offer the courses simultaneously, in a process that is often referred to as "stacking." We used two adjoining classrooms (one a studio for group work, the other a classroom with tables, chairs, and learning technologies) and team-taught.

To solve the problem of students needing separate curricular information and attention, we developed the course as hybrids — students and instructors met *together* weekly and again in separate online modules.[4] Playwriting students had the opportunity to work on a specific skill set (like writing a scene or dialogue), while Storytelling students could work on oral history. Playwriting focused on using the ethnographic material, experience, and transcripts collected by Storytelling groups at Luther Manor. They also wrote scripted presentations that dramatized the material. The culminating capstone project (written plays and scenarios) was a celebration at Luther Manor in mid-December, which served as a primer to the Sojourn production that would be staged the following March. Despite the compression of schedules and use of online systems, transportation and scheduling still proved to be one of the more challenging aspects of the classes. Curricular goals for the Storytelling students included learning to invite stories from people with disabilities; learning to create and facilitate their own storytelling group sessions; learning to document, code, and analyze collected stories as data; and learning how to respectfully and insightfully perform stories back to the people from whom they were originally gathered. At least one Playwriting student served on each of the Storytelling teams that dispersed throughout Luther Manor. Curricular goals for the Playwriting students included learning basic plot and story structure and learning to gather stories as data and transform it into short plays.

While university administration encourages innovative teaching (like sharing courses and materials), the practice has little structural support. The university mechanisms for assigning instruction, tracking the profitability of courses, locating courses in classrooms, and so forth are all set up to encourage one teacher per class — isolated from others and separated in subjects or fields of study. The fact that we prevailed in our collaboration — and succeeded — is testimony to our perseverance and support of each other. There were several times we could easily have walked away from offering Penelope courses as a block because the validity of the work was frequently challenged and questioned by our peers.

On Thursday afternoons, students would arrive at a bus stop on a corner near campus where a Luther Manor bus would meet and take them to their site. For two hours students worked collaboratively with group members on exploring and expressing Penelope's story — in relation to their own. The remaining half hour at Luther Manor was a debriefing and a bus trip back to campus. Throughout the semester, Storytelling and Playwriting students were required to work collaboratively with Luther Manor staff and residents in small groups and to create a final presentation that was inclusive of all group members. These groups were identified by their location and level of service to residents: the Courtyards (assisted living), the Day Center, the Health Care Center (skilled nursing), and the Terrace (independent living) groups. Each group was overseen by the activities and program coordinators assigned to these areas, who discovered that the process was really about co-learning. This excerpt from a Luther Manor staff email reveals both the planning and the feelings about the process:

> Tuesday the UWM professors, Sojourn Theatre, and Luther Manor
> team met during the lunch hour, to review the project, tell stories, learn
> about each other, and validate our individual talents. We are also being
> encouraged to create ideas and input, track our feelings and emotions —

the sublime, upsetting, and the exuberant. We learned that the students who are coming are not all in art or theatre. They are studying storytelling to learn about themselves and our elders. It was a valuable time for me personally because we are encouraged to assist the UWM students in this learning experiment.

Every Tuesday afternoon, students and instructors would meet on campus to review, explore new concepts, and plan the work together. The students' Class Reports that follow give a sense of how the students shaped their sessions, including exercises that they learned in class and how they adjusted to what they were discovering.

Class Report: The 8-Week Plan Report
Week 1: We have nametags for everyone (as per M's suggestion, the residents can decorate them and we've got art supplies). We also have an introductory ice-breaker game to learn names. Then we'll discuss aspects of the Penelope story and have activities based on those themes. We'll close with saying a quick thing about what we all learned or liked about today and what we want to learn or talk about next time.
Class Report:
Week 3 Check-in: We've got some suggestions — and we are checking in on how things have been going. This group has been thinking about Penelope a lot and having discussion about "doing a play" and about acting. [We want] to review what they are doing and how they envision their role. We want to do some acting exercises — so that is planned. Also, some of the group members have been at Luther Manor for over 10 years. We have been hearing advice from them. And we will do role-playing.

The end of semester performance of original stories took place in the Faith and Education Center at Luther Manor in mid-December 2010. Residents, staff, and volunteers from all four areas of care assembled for the program. Sojourn Theatre artists from Chicago attended, as did students who had been involved with the previous semester's research efforts. In total, approximately two hundred people attended. Basting and Beth Meyer-Arnold introduced the overall project, and UWM classics professor Andrew Porter made a brief and popular presentation on Greek epic poetry, the story of Penelope, and a bit about ancient Greek culture, including teaching the diverse audience how to sing the Greek alphabet.

The final course attached to the Penelope Project was Theatre 475: Performance Workshop, offered in the spring 2011 semester. Anne Basting was the instructor of record for this course—a practice-based, credit-bearing option for those students who were assigned as assistant director, assistant dramaturge, assistant stage manager, cast, or crew. Together, the pre-research project, the jointly offered Storytelling and Playwriting courses, and the Performance Workshop provided a three-semester sequence that involved seventy-five UWM students for credit. Most students were involved for only one of the three semesters, enabling them to cycle in and out as their intense credit loads and rigid department course of study demanded. While the project had a specific overarching goal (to improve the quality of life for all those who live in, work in, and visit Luther Manor), student goals depended on the curricular framework for the course in which they were enrolled. As educators engaged in the overarching project, we sought to improve the quality of life of the students by bringing them into meaningful engagement with older adults, some of whom had significant disabilities. In the final section of the book, we describe how we went about evaluating our success on this front, through a series of pre- and post-surveys and through analyzing student field notes and reflections throughout the various semesters.

NOTES

1. Designed and taught by Dr. Basting in 2006.
2. Designed and taught by Dr. Mello in 2007 and 2008.
3. Designed and taught by Dr. Mello in 2005.
4. For a detailed description of the course(s), goals, and calendar, see appendix 5.

THE STRUCTURE AND EVOLUTION OF FUNDING FOR PENELOPE

Anne Basting

Over my fifteen years in working in the arts with health care systems, I have affirmed my original intuition — that if you invite creative expression, you need to value it and show others (staff, family, other residents, the outside world) that it has value. That takes time, effort, and high-quality supplies. It takes artistic rigor, and rigor costs money.

How did we go about planning the budget and support of this mammoth project? First, the partners all assumed financial responsibility for the project. In the opening phase of the project, we created a partnership agreement document in which each partnering organization identified one common goal for the project along with a series of objectives unique to that organization. Each organization stated clearly, in bullet-point form, what it would commit to as part of the project. This included supporting other organizations to achieve their objectives and assisting in raising funds for the project as a whole. (Note: The partnership agreement is included in the appendix.) To raise a significant amount of funds for the project, we would need to look to places that would fund only the artistic component — and Sojourn would lead on those grants. We would need to look to funds that would support only community organizations or, even more specifically, Lutheran organizations. Luther Manor would be the lead on and receiver of those funds. And there would be sources that only the university would be eligible to receive or that UWM had the strongest chance of receiving due to the research and educational base of the institution. I created and shared a template proposal that would serve as the base for adaptations to a wide variety of foundations to which the team applied for funding. Our eventual budget for the project was an elaborate chart that monitored multiple sources submitted by three different entities over multiple years. The budget in itself was a work of art.

Second, we agreed from the beginning that the project should aim for the highest quality on all fronts — in performance, education, research/evaluation, and documentation. We all agreed that this balance should be reflected in our funding sources, so we actively sought out funding in the various program areas — arts, education, social services. We aimed for the funding portfolio to be an endorsement of the quality of the project on all fronts. A high-quality arts project that receives only social service funding risks being perceived mainly as a social service project. Our diverse funding portfolio would be an integral part of our project description.

Third, we needed to financially support all phases of the project, from development to dissemination, with equal time, money, and effort. Partnership development, preliminary research, creative experimentation, and the final artistic production are all equally integral parts of the project. To "go cheap" on any of them would be to devalue its role in the process.

Fourth, we needed to be sure that all partners felt supported, whether it was in-kind time or paid time from the project. Resentment among partners, no matter how engaged they are or how exciting the project is, would be toxic to collaboration.

We never imagined that the project would be replicable by others on the same scale. Because we wanted to create teaching and dissemination tools to come from a project that had never been tried before, we had significant additional costs that others can be spared.

We aimed to make the project sustainable by integrating it into the daily workload/life of the participants so that after the funding receded, it would be possible to continue on to the next creative project at Luther Manor. Because programming staff at Luther Manor had to do programming anyway, we imagined that staff could continue with additional projects. But it proved crucial to have the buy-in from administrators for programming staff to take the extra time this first project demanded. The project was, indeed, larger than any project that would come after it, and it demanded logistical details that other projects might not, including consent forms from staff and residents (to be involved in research and to use their image and creative expression in the play and promotional materials); recruitment of participants; management of parking, security, transportation, public relations, and ticket sales; and so forth.

Also with an eye on sustainability, Robin Mello and I integrated our time through existing university funding structures, namely teaching and administration. Our time was supported partially by grants but mostly by integrating the project into our teaching duties. I had additional support of my time from my 50 percent administrative position as director of the Center on Age & Community (CAC). CAC administered the funds from the Helen Bader Foundation, the Brookdale Foundation, and Wisconsin Representatives of Activity Professionals and funds derived from the training fees from TimeSlips Creative Storytelling. Sojourn Theatre administered funds from the MAP Fund. Luther Manor administered funds from the Wisconsin Humanities Council, Wisconsin Arts Board, and several small grants/gifts. In conference calls with key staff from each partnering organization, we managed logistics for this complex funding structure. At project's end, I created a general report that could be adapted to grant reports by all three partnering organizations.

See the appendix for a full list of funding partners and a description of their role in supporting the project.

THE STRUCTURE AND EVOLUTION
OF EVALUATION OF PENELOPE
Anne Basting

All partners agreed that we needed to wrap meaningful evaluation around Penelope to understand what was changing for all players, including students, staff, residents, artists, family, and volunteers. Understanding the impact of the project would help us better design future projects and legitimize community-engaged practice in teaching and artistic practice in the eyes of participants, partners, and potential funders. Committing to rigorous evaluation, however, demands considerable advance planning and effort. My position as director of the UWM Center on Age & Community made this extensive evaluation process possible.

CAC post-doc fellow Jason Danely worked with me to write and submit a human subjects protocol to UWM's Institutional Review Board (IRB). Any research that focuses on human subjects must follow strict guidelines and be approved by the IRB. This meant that we had to create, distribute, and track consent forms for the many participants in the project, including students, staff, older adults, older adults with cognitive disabilities, volunteers, and artists. To simplify this complicated process, we created a single, universal consent form for the many components of the project. This universal consent form covered permission to use photographs, sound, video, and any artwork participants might create in the project. It also asked permission to conduct interviews, focus groups, and surveys. The consent process for residents and participants at Luther Manor took considerable time and was generously coordinated by staff at Luther Manor. Even without the research study, however, the fact that we were sharing the residents' creative input and documenting the process in video and audio recording and still photography would have demanded that we secure consents. We gathered consents on a rolling basis — whenever new people joined the project, they were offered a consent form, even if they joined the project the week before the play opened.

We designed a similar consent form for students that specifically addressed the fact that they could choose *not* to participate in the study and still fully participate in the class. If they did agree to participate in the study, all their assignments would be considered data and could be used in the final program evaluation. We would supply them with a pseudonym to protect their identity if we used their work in any publications.

We designed a third consent form for Sojourn artists. Similarly, the artists agreed to do interviews and focus groups, to take pre- and post-surveys, and that all artistic process and product could be considered as data.

What were we looking for the evaluation to show? What impact did we hope to measure? Part of our research was exploratory. Nothing of this scale had been tried before. We didn't know what impact we might have, so we wrapped qualitative interviews and focus groups around the projects to observe, listen, and learn how people described the impact in their own words. We imagined that the project would change people's perspectives about working with older adults with disabilities. There is a workforce crisis brewing in this country because of negative assumptions about careers working with older adults and because of low-wages associated with their care. While we couldn't impact pay scale, we hoped we could improve attitudes. We used pre- and post-surveys of student, artist, and staff attitudes toward working with older adults with disabilities to see if collaborative art-making could change these deeply engrained attitudes that working with older adults is "depressing" or, at worst, futile. This survey had been used by other researchers and shown to be a "valid" instrument to measure attitudes. We offered the survey to participants at the beginning of their involvement in the project and again at the end. The survey is included in the appendix of the book, as are sample consent forms. We also designed an online survey that was emailed to audience members who attended the play. All our notes from meetings with the key staff and project leaders also became data to inform our understanding of how the project unfolded and what impact it had. We held several official focus group meetings after key stages of the project, including one with Storytelling and Playwriting students after their fall semester; one with the artists after the completion of the play; one with staff/family/residents after the completion of the play; and one with a group of experts that we invited to attend the final performance of the play.

HIPAA (Health Insurance Portability and Accountability Act) regulations and requirements demanded that we train the artists and students not to reveal private medical information about any Luther Manor participants. Similarly, FERPA (Family Educational Rights and Privacy Act) demanded that we shape the evaluation in a way that protected the identity of the students.

TABLE 1. PROGRAM EVALUATION DATA MATRIX

PENELOPE PROJECT

Constituents	Participant observations[1]	Interviews, blogs, and emails[2]	Visual data[3]	Artifacts[4]	Surveys
Artists	x	x	x	x	x
Staff and faculty connected with ST, CAC, UWM, DT, and LM	x	x	x	x	
UWM students		x	x	x	x
Audiences		x	x		x
Family and friends		x	x		x
FP chorus	x	x	x		x
LM residents	x		x	x	x

CAC: Center on Age & Community
DT: Department of Theatre
FP: *Finding Penelope* (the play)
LM: Luther Manor
ST: Sojourn Theatre
UWM: University of Wisconsin–Milwaukee

Notes
1. These include classes, seminars, meetings, work sessions, TimeSlips sessions, rehearsals, workshops, performances, and conferences.
2. These include face-to-face and computer-mediated interviews, phone conferences, focus groups, transcripts of these interview data, etc.
3. These include video and film recordings, transcripts of video and film recordings, photographs, etc.
4. These include art projects, weaving, songs, poems, flyers, notes, maps, drafts of plays, diaries, logs, internal memos, emails, text messages, photographs, webpages, blogs, students' written and digital assignments, course evaluations, grant narratives, etc.

At project's end, my colleague Robin Mello gathered all data and conducted a full program evaluation. In some ways, our creative research could also be described as process evaluation — measuring our progress against the goals and objectives we had set out in our partnership agreements at the very beginning of the project. We used the regular stakeholder meetings to understand how we could better help each partner achieve their objectives, and then we adjusted to improve our practice. Mello's final program evaluation looks at our original objectives and observes what actually happened — identifying key characteristics/philosophies of the project that guided our steps. Excerpts from the program evaluation and a description of its methodology appear in part five. The chart shows all the data that we gathered and used to inform our conclusions about the impact of the project.

THE MYTHIC LENS OF PENELOPE
Robin Mello and Anne Basting

ANNE

When I was first contemplating how to embed Penelope into the Department of Theatre at UWM, I made a date with my colleague Robin Mello to talk through my ideas. A year earlier, when the department staged Barbara Ehrenreich's *Nickel and Dimed*, Mello had done an original play devised from interviews her students gathered about living on minimum wage in Milwaukee. When I sat down with her and told her about my idea — to create a play inspired by the story of Penelope from the *Odyssey* — she got a funny look on her face. "You know I did my dissertation on Penelope and female heroes, don't you?" No, in fact, I didn't. Robin became a fountain of knowledge about the power of mythic structures and how they function differently for male and female characters. We also worked closely with Andrew Porter, a classics scholar at UWM, to unlock some of the language and historical context of the *Odyssey*. Why use myth? What is its unique power? Robin tells us in the essay that follows.

ROBIN

Myths are stories that help us make sense of our world and are awash with elemental forces, generative energies, and monsters engaged in life-or-death struggles. Myths illustrate human fears, values, and beliefs. The hero of myth is a character who struggles with his humanity. He struggles to make difficult choices, especially when the odds are stacked against him. Mythic heroes are imperfect and mortal, just as we are.

Myths — especially hero tales, with their monsters and insurmountable obstacles — illustrate the human condition in larger-than-life ways. The story of Penelope and Odysseus is one of those myths that gives us a view into human joy and suffering. Their story also provides us with an opportunity to balance mythological values and actions against our own. The story of Queen Penelope's efforts to preserve her honor and her son's life becomes an elevated drama that allows us to admire and aspire toward greatness — to be like her. Hearing about Penelope's and Odysseus' hardships allows us to empathize with their condition and imagine ourselves in their place. We get to set ourselves on the throne of Ithaca, borrow their cunning, participate in their dilemmas, and link real and mythical worlds together.

Connecting myths from different world cultures together—then framing them into formulas, character types, and structures—is an idea that has been around for at least a century. Jung, Freud, Bly, and Campbell, to name a few, used mythic patterns and archetypes to contextualize human psychological and developmental processes. Penelope's story, within the *Odyssey*, is one of these archetypes.

The Penelope Project used myth as a context and metaphor, which specifically helped explore the status and condition of people living in long-term care. Penelope is a heroine, a feminine hero—very different from her husband, Odysseus. She is not part of the masculine hero story of world myth (for example, Maui, Hercules, or King Arthur). Penelope's power lies in the fact that she is a mother, wife, queen, and keeper of traditions. Heroines like Penelope are a counterpoint to the role that mythic heroes play in stories. Her story balances the macro-myth and provides an alternative to the swashbuckling he-man conqueror of hero tales.

Importantly, Penelope, like many other mythic heroines, is not a warrior. She doesn't wield a sword or do battle with monsters (although one could count the hordes of suitors who have taken advantage of her hospitality as monstrous). Instead of violently confronting Ithaca's invaders, she waits, watches, and employs cunning diplomacy while she weaves and unweaves a delicate linen shroud so detailed and refined that it conceivably just *might* actually take ten years to complete. Because of her disinclination to confront her Achaean guests openly (as her husband and son do toward the end of the *Odyssey*), she has often been thought of as a bit of a wimp, a whiner, a powerless character who is waiting to be "saved" by a man. Nothing could be further from the truth. Penelope is a symbol of perseverance, loyalty, and power.

Other valuable but sometimes overlooked characteristics are Penelope's ethical stance and beauty. She is challenged numerous times to take the easy way out, but she chooses the honorable, more difficult path instead. Her great beauty is important—as it represents her innate power and quality of character, but it is both a blessing and a curse. Still, she uses it chastely and humanely. Penelope's decision to remain faithful to her husband is clearly emphasized when Homer, in the *Odyssey*, balances Penelope's actions against that of Queen Clytemnestra who does take a lover while King Agamemnon is away at war. Clytemnestra is decidedly not a heroine, nor does she share a heroine's fate. In comparison Penelope rises.

Yet, our popular cultural media is full of the classic male adventurer — so much so that the hero archetype is often held up as the *only* example of bravery and courage. Unfortunately, this also means that we have less balance in our cultural mythic imagination. We have limited our creative options and also cut ourselves off from honoring alternative experiences. From *Dungeons & Dragons* to the *Game of Thrones* and from *Star Wars* to *X-Men*, storytellers in the entertainment industry keep recycling the ancient mythic pattern of the hero's journey. People love heroes. The traditional hero model, or mythic cycle, goes something like this: A man, Odysseus for example, starts out as a loner; he is an orphan and born to royalty. One day, our hero is suddenly called out of obscurity and told that great things are expected of him. He is forced to leave home and endures years of hardship, battle, and conflict. He kills monsters and when he does also loses almost everyone and everything that he loves. Eventually he returns home to settle down and becomes a wise and just ruler. This is Harry Potter, Superman, Spiderman, Bilbo, Wolverine, and Luke Skywalker's story. The list goes on and on. But there is *another* mythic model out there, one just as dynamic but much less famous. It is the heroine's story.

Who and what is a mythic heroine? Her name is Penelope, Deirdre of the Sorrows, Gudrun, Shiva, Scheherazade, and Ruth, to name a few. The heroine plot goes something like this: She's an orphan, or a daughter of a king, who is so beautiful that it is apparent from the very day of her birth that she is destined for great or unusual things. As she grows up, many men try to woo her and/or own her, but she refuses all suitors and chooses, instead, a husband of her liking (he is often a hero). At this point she is banished from her home and forced to live in exile. Then, through a long series of difficulties, the mythic heroine becomes separated from her husband and/or children, imprisoned, isolated, and often enslaved. She is publically humiliated and shamed (there are many heroine myths where she is left to live in the streets and forced to beg for her food in order to stay alive), yet she remains steadfast and strong. In the end, she is vindicated, reunited with her family, and reigns as queen.

While the hero story is a cycle, the heroine myth tends to be iterative. The plot repeats itself in a kind of spiral that winds around and back again. Heroes encounter one thing after another. In a hero story, a dragon might appear, and when it is vanquished our hero might confront a giant troll, and so on. In heroine stories things don't happen in such a linear fashion. For example, Penelope endures ten years of waiting for news of Odysseus' fate while he is away at war. Then, finally, news arrives — the Greeks are victorious. What happens then? Ten more years of waiting.

We overlook the fact that heroines are often vilified and imprisoned for long periods of time (like Penelope's twenty-year vigil). Their options are often more limited than a hero's. On the other hand, a heroine's limitations often turn out to be opportunities in disguise. In the book of Ruth, for example, the heroine uses hardship as inspiration to convert to Judaism and, in so doing, preserves an entire culture and way of life. In fact, preservation of home and family are important tasks given almost exclusively to heroines. Unfortunately, heroines of myth, like Penelope, have, over time, been written out of their own stories and have become almost invisible. In working on the Penelope Project, we were able to explore and reclaim her.

Penelope became the project's mythic frame as well as its identity. We explored the important dynamics embedded in her story, investigating experiences such as giving birth, keeping families together, raising children, growing old, and facing death alone. We found connections to Penelope's condition both at Luther Manor and at UWM. Students and Luther Manor residents related to our mythic heroine because they, like Penelope, often experience being overlooked, undervalued, or limited in their resources and options. They rely on inner resources and must remain steadfast in the face of adversity. During this project we had an opportunity not only to make Penelope visible but also to update her for the contemporary moment. We found that she is still as vital, viable, and pertinent as she was to Greek audiences in 800 BCE.

PART THREE: *Resistance, Realizations, and Adjustments*

Penelope was an iterative project that grew through collaboration. Together, the three core partners (Luther Manor, UWM, and Sojourn Theatre) had a shared goal and an imagined path. As we set out on our path, myriad challenges and realities popped up. In essence, we had committed to not knowing what would happen—and to step forward by communicating and adjusting as the project evolved. This was not easy for staff members who work in a system of regulation and routine. It was not easy for students, whose grades depend on them clearly understanding what is expected. It was easiest for the artists, who were used to this improvisational mode of working, but the new and unique challenges of working in a hyper-regulated long-term care setting clogged their confidence and caused some serious second-guessing. This section focuses on those myriad challenges, the learning moments, and the adjustments we all made as we moved forward.

EXCERPT FROM *Finding Penelope*, SCENE 1
Anne Basting

Scene 1: In the lobby of the Faith and Education Center—poised to enter the nursing home

OLD BEGGAR *walks forward, but* MIRA *stops, clinging to the handrail for dear life.*

OLD BEGGAR
Aren't you coming?

MIRA
I—I—I can't—I just can't—

OLD BEGGAR
It appears to be—a hallway. I see no monsters. . . . What is there to fear?
(*This is an earnest question.*)

MIRA
I'm afraid I'm afraid to say.

CHORUS
SHE'S AFRAID SHE'S AFRAID TO SAY.

OLD BEGGAR
Are you afraid of your *mother?*

MIRA
No. Maybe. I'm afraid of—I'm embarrassed to say it.

OLD BEGGAR
You must name it to slay it.

MIRA
I'm afraid I'm afraid of—the smell.

CHORUS
SHE'S AFRAID SHE'S AFRAID OF THE SMELL.

MIRA
Shhhh! Don't repeat that! They'll hear!

CHORUS

SHHHH! DON'T REPEAT THAT! WE'LL HEAR!

OLD BEGGAR

Dear Mira. Nothing, but nothing smells as putrid as the rotting carcasses of a 1,000 young soldiers piled up within the walls of Troy. Except perhaps me. (*noting his rags*) Or your imagination. This place? Fresh as an ocean breeze. Off we go then to find Penelope.

CHORUS

OUR CUNNING, NOBLE, WISE, AND LOVELY QUEEN!

OLD BEGGAR moves forward. MIRA scoots down the handrail and clings to it dearly. OLD BEGGAR sees her retreat and is on guard.

OLD BEGGAR

What is it? What do you see?

MIRA

I'm afraid someone will cry — that someone will cry out for help — and I won't know what to do.

CHORUS

SHE'S AFRAID WE'LL CRY AND SHE WON'T KNOW WHAT TO DO.

MIRA

I'm afraid I'm afraid of the icy fingers of death.

CHORUS

WEAR A COAT.

OLD BEGGAR

That's a good idea. I would give you mine but I'm afraid it's a bit soiled.

MIRA

I'm afraid I'm afraid of the guilt.

OLD BEGGAR

Ah. Yes. I know it well. But I don't believe it is lethal.

MIRA

I'm afraid I'm afraid I'm afraid I'm afraid I'm afraid.

CHORUS

WE ARE ALL AFRAID. ALWAYS AND EVERYWHERE.

MIRA

I'm afraid I'm afraid it will happen to me.

CHORUS

DON'T BE AFRAID, MIRA. THE STRANGE, OLD BEGGAR WHO LOOKS
NOTHING LIKE ODYSSEUS WILL HELP YOU.

OLD BEGGAR

Well, I don't have a good track record of keeping my colleagues alive. But I
promise I will protect you.

ON FEAR AND TREPIDATION

Anne Basting

"I work in aging."
PAUSE (no response)

I encounter that PAUSE on a daily basis. Predictably, it follows my response to questions like "What do you do?" But it also follows my question to social work students, nursing and medical students, even emerging artists:

"Have you ever thought about working with older adults?"
PAUSE

That pause is quite full. Research on stereotypes tells us that we associate older people with being "warm" but "incompetent" (Cuddy, Norton, and Fisk 2005). Terror management research tells us that young people in particular find the mere mention of aging, disability, and death to be significant triggers for stress (Greenberg 2012). That stigma can be carried into the workplace. Professional fields such as social work, nursing, dentistry, and medicine have a difficult time recruiting students (Lee et al. 2013). One can peer into the pause and see what causes it pretty clearly. Fear of disability. Fear of aging. Fear of mortality. Fear of not earning enough to pay back college loans. Fear of working in a "depressing" job.

Unexamined fear breeds avoidance. And that is where we are with aging in the United States. We avoid talking about it. We avoid doing anything about how to fund caring for it. We avoid actually *doing* it — or appearing to do it — if we can afford to. The marks of time on the body are equated with a lack of money or ability to erase them.

In many ways, the Penelope Project was an invitation to examine those fears in order to imagine an end to avoidance and connect across generations and abilities. When Robin Mello and I combined our Playwriting and Storytelling classes, we gave students a survey in the beginning of class that assessed their attitudes toward aging in general and disabilities like dementia in particular. We worked with students in the classroom for several weeks before going out to Luther Manor to meet our partners. We told stories about older people in our lives. We examined our fears of mortality, of disability, of aging. Robin led a particularly powerful exercise called the "Elder Circle" in which students lined up in order of age and then formed a circle. Starting with the youngest person, each student said something he or she learned about life so far and asked a question about life that he or she hadn't yet understood or figured out. Each person asked that question of the person in front of him or her—the next-oldest person. The comments and questions ranged from entertaining to profound. The final moment was the most moving. The oldest person in the group asked a question of the youngest person, who was the start of the circle. "How do I parent a child who is at college? I want to show him I care and can help, but I don't want to crowd him." The youngest person responded, "I would ask him that exact question. I bet he will tell you."

The students also wrote journal entries and field notes that detailed what Robin and I (and the residents and staff) could see from the outside—that as the semester wore on, they paused less and engaged more. Their post-surveys revealed the same. The journey away from fear and avoidance was so pronounced that we made it the story of the play itself. Two characters serve as our guides through the play. Odysseus, disguised as an old beggar, is freshly home after twenty years. He is afraid that Penelope has forgotten him. Mira is the daughter of a (made-up) resident in the assisted living area of Luther Manor. A rocky relationship with her mother and her fears of long-term care kept her away for twenty years. In the opening scene Mira relays her fears, only to be cajoled by an unseen chorus. When Odysseus asks her why she won't go into the nursing area, she responds, "I'm afraid I'm afraid to say." "I'm afraid I'm afraid of—the smell," she confesses, only to have it echoed more loudly by the chorus: "She's afraid she's afraid of the smell." "Shhhh," she pleads. "They'll hear." "Shhhh," they echo. "We'll hear." Finally, she sheepishly admits, "I'm afraid it will happen to me." "Don't be afraid, Mira," affirms the chorus. "The strange, old beggar who looks nothing like Odysseus will help you." And together, guided by musicians singing "Sentimental Journey," they walk into the nursing home on their journey to find Penelope. Aristotle writes, in translation, that tragedy is the purgation of pity and fear. *Finding Penelope* shared that goal but also sought to disarm fears with a healthy dose of humor.

The PAUSE comes from the other side of the age spectrum too—both from the staff and from the older adults themselves. Their fears triggering avoidance were not so different from those of the younger students. In continuing care communities, it is not uncommon for people in independent senior apartments to stop visiting their friends when they move to either assisted living or skilled nursing where disability can be an uncomfortable reminder of what might lie ahead for them. One of our objectives with Penelope was to foster connection among staff and residents across the great divides among care areas. We were surprised to realize that programming staff had never collaborated across areas before Penelope. And after Penelope, this would prove to be one of the ongoing challenges for Luther Manor — to maintain the collaboration across areas when budgeting, reporting, job descriptions/evaluations, and sheer square footage (Luther Manor is a million square feet) encourage silos.

Why exactly do young people avoid engaging with older people? Why avoid work that might bring you into contact with older people? Why do older people avoid other older people with disabilities? Why do staff avoid the possibilities yielded by collaboration, or the possibilities of longer-term projects rather than activities that don't grow over time? Research offers psychological clues to the answer to these questions that are rolled into fears of mortality and disability. But at the end of the day, I think it might simply be that at heart, people don't want to hurt each other's feelings. "I'm afraid I will say the wrong thing," wrote more than one student to explain fears of engaging with older people. Just how does one be in company with people that one perceives as sad or suffering? One cheers them up with a game of bingo. Or one avoids them entirely. One becomes "too busy" to listen and share a moment together. We seem to find it very difficult to believe that there can be joy comingled in the challenges of aging and/or disability. In the presence of loss, we find it impossible to see anything else. And so we continue the cycle. Fear. Avoidance. PAUSE.

WORKS CITED

Cuddy, Amy J. C., Michael I. Norton, and Susan T. Fiske. 2005. "This Old Stereotype: The Pervasiveness and Persistence of the Elderly Stereotype." *Journal of Social Issues* 61 (2): 267–85.

Greenberg, Jeff. 2012. "Terror Management Theory: From Genesis to Revelations." In *Meaning, Mortality, and Choice: The Social Psychology of Existential Concerns*, edited by Phillip R. Shaver and Mario Mikulincer, 17–35. Washington, DC: American Psychological Association.

Lee, Wei-Chen, et al. 2013. "Meeting the Geriatric Workforce Shortage for Long-Term Care: Opinions from the Field." *Gerontology & Geriatrics Education* 34 (4): 354–71.

STAFF RESISTANCES, REACTIONS, AND INTERACTIONS
Ellie Rose

Project director Anne Basting and Luther Manor staff liaison Beth Meyer-Arnold introduced the Penelope Project to Luther Manor staff during standard monthly meetings, such as our third-Wednesday-of-the-month Management Council meeting, with both administrative and life enrichment staff invited. They described Penelope as an invitation for all people living in, working in, and visiting Luther Manor to take part in an arts project in any way they wanted. This meant we, as managers and programming staff, were expected to involve the residents, staff, and caregivers in each of our care areas. Staff members brought up concerns and questions about the uncertainty of the outcomes. There were concerns of safety, regulations, and heartfelt ideals that it is our responsibility to anticipate the needs of the residents. I wondered what it meant to anticipate people's needs. Did it mean that if people spilled tea on their shirt once that they would forever after need to wear a "clothing protector" (also known as a bib)? I heard things like "My people won't like that" and "My people aren't able to do that." Sad and discouraged, I found myself screaming in my head, "Really? Not one person has the ability to engage in an open creative project that has no restrictions?"

In April 2010, Sojourn and UWM offered an eight-hour training workshop at Luther Manor for select staff. We were invited to read an interpretation of the *Odyssey* before attending the training and could join in the retelling of the story if we wanted. Penelope Project artists facilitated discussions to gather ideas of the meaning, purpose, and logistics of the project. They also guided the group through a variety of creative engagement techniques. Among the staff, immediate responses to the training were, "How are we going to invite others to be involved?" and "What are we required to offer in addition to our already busy activity schedules?" In so many minds, Penelope seemed like it was going to be a lot of extra work.

Over lunch we discussed the need for monthly meetings and weekly check-ins, the various deadlines, and the expectations of some kind of product to come from the project. We were going to need to find ways to share our schedules, shift our routine activities, and share our progress. How were we going to effectively communicate when some of us rarely have the time to check our email?

Some of us staff were excited to finally have the chance to work together. For example, one of the independent living life enrichment specialists and I had been trying to work on a project together for months with little success. Our schedules never matched, and residents were committed to their routines. The demand of other activities, our personal work schedules, and transportation needs suffocated our visions of partnering. We needed something more to make it happen. Penelope empowered our activity programs to change. We had a reason, even a requirement, to change because management and administration were on board. It was like receiving a gold baton to conduct an orchestra of creative people we engaged with every day.

During and after that first Penelope training, it was clear that collaboration wasn't going to be easy, nor should it have been. Meaning and purpose do not bloom from isolation and routine, and there is risk with change. Resident safety would have to be observed instead of expected, and regulations would have to be analyzed instead of followed to the letter. It was going to take energy and rigor.

Person-centered care and relationship building were the core of all of our programs, so it wasn't difficult to figure out where to start. We talked with our staff teams and resident small groups about Odysseus and Penelope. A volunteer shared her story about true love, and a resident spoke of what it was like to be away from his wife during the war. A staff person overheard a conversation and interrupted to share her definition of home, and a resident followed her story with a defiant outcry, "Home is where your family is. If you don't have your family, you have nothing!"

This engagement in storytelling and themes from the student discussions helped us to overcome the staff's focus on attendance — judging the success of a program by how many people show. Many of the students had little experience in care settings, and I found myself educating them about how to engage with older adults, especially those living with dementia. They needed education in how to gather a small group, how to guide a conversation instead of lead it, and how to assist others with physical and cognitive challenges. It was powerful to feel the residents, students, and staff all learning and sharing together. Bingo couldn't do that.

In the months that followed we reshaped our existing program of activities to include Penelope by changing the focus and titles of our activities. We offered collaborative projects like the Penelope Weaving and the Penelope Welcome Dance that would have otherwise been run as "Crocheting" and "Morning Movements." The independent care area offered activities like the Health Care Center's Penelope Tea and the Adult Day Center's Origami Love Letters (in which residents wrote letters between Penelope and Odysseus and then folded them into origami birds), previously known as "Tea Time" and "Poetry Corner."

Despite the success in some Penelope activities, there were moments of staff doubt and resistance to change. There were complaints of the extensive preparation for some activities and the additional time required in completing projects, like Penelope's mural. Two months into the project I began journaling because I was struggling to make sense of the challenges. Penelope meetings turned into places for complaining and confusion. In one conversation between three care areas, one staff member refused to participate in the weaving. There were too many expectations, and Penelope often took away from traditional activities like Bible Study on Thursdays and Coffee Talk on Monday mornings. The meeting ended with this bold statement: "My people don't understand Penelope, and dementia people cannot weave!" It was obvious the staff had low expectations of the residents and did not understand the deeper intentions of Penelope. It was not the individuals living with dementia that were unable to weave; rather the staff members were not using or creating strategies to support them in doing it.

During their residency, Sojourn Theatre and UWM staff and students were everywhere at Luther Manor. At first they would meet in a conference room because Wi-Fi was crucial, but then they started having meetings in random hallways and even took screens off and crawled out windows for dramatic effects in the play. Many department heads and nursing staff were just plain frustrated with the "Penelope People" (as they called them) because they were "interfering" with their tasks and responsibilities. For example, the actors were laughing in nursing areas and inviting residents to join in conversation during what is normally a nap time after lunch. When they got lost, staff and residents would have to redirect them, and if they had questions, we stopped to answer them. The best part of working with them was teaching them that Luther Manor was not only a place to visit but a living, breathing community on which they were having an impact every day they were there.

With so much staff resistance to this "home invasion," why did we continue? Because the benefits were radiating from the residents' faces, and because the community, the larger society — the outside world — needed to hear them, and it became our responsibility to offer opportunities for the residents to express themselves, take action, and be heard.

CHALLENGES FOR STUDENTS
Robin Mello

To engage students in the Penelope Project, Basting and I created a sequence of three courses over three semesters. The first was a research course in which students provided background research on the *Odyssey* and helped shape a project guide to help with explaining the project to students, elders, staff, and family. The second was really two courses, Storytelling and Playwriting, in which students would lead creative discussions at Luther Manor. The third was for students engaged in the performance of *Finding Penelope*, as actors, assistant directors, and assistant designers. This essay focuses on the unique challenges of the Storytelling and Playwriting courses.

Creating a classroom in the community, also known as "engaged learning," is a powerful experience for students, community members, and faculty alike. But students also faced challenges — and considerable rewards — inside these "engaged" class structures. The Penelope courses were built out of regular Department of Theatre offerings at UWM. Most students take these courses to meet an arts requirement (the university requires arts credits in all degree programs). Other students enrolled because these courses are required electives within the major (BA theatre degree), and a few simply because the course content sounded interesting to them. At the start we had approximately twenty students. Most felt that they were in for "an easy A," likely thinking, "How difficult could a class on storytelling be?"

This "engaged" classroom experience was a bit different from others on campus. Most engaged classes include community partnerships that are contained within the boundaries of that single semester. This class would be part of a much larger project that was "iterative" — or open-ended. The students would have a part in shaping the overall project, but we couldn't describe fully what Penelope would become because it was evolving as the extensive partnerships continued to grow. So the students' first surprise came during the initial introductory overview. We excitedly presented our research and vision (which at that time was almost all we had) and the proposed work plan (which was admittedly heavy and complicated). There were many surprised faces when these undergraduates discovered we were inviting them to participate in a unique community project that was going to send them off campus and seemed to have no clearly defined end point — with the exception of a project at the end of the semester that would eventually inform the play that Sojourn Theatre would create together in January.

Students expressed resistance immediately. But, at this point, it was a function of them adjusting their expectations and trying to conceptualize, in a concrete way, what the project might actually feel and look like. Despite the open-ended scope of the plan, the students' curiosity was engaged. We challenged them. They, in turn, adjusted their expectations. Resistance gave way to enthusiasm.

As the semester went on, games, storytelling and playwriting practices, and improvisations (like telling/acting out the *Odyssey* in under fifteen minutes) created cohesion. A visit from UWM classics professor Andrew Porter gave the students confidence in their understanding of Penelope's story and the cultural context of the work. A visit from Luther Manor's Beth Meyer-Arnold began to build bridges to the long-term care community. The class experience was motivating and rewarding. Online, at our course website, we required students to work in planning groups where they formulated strategies and wrote sample scripts that would be used toward their eventual exploration of Penelope's story at Luther Manor. Overall, during this phase, our students brought joy and energy to the project, and we got to see concrete evidence that our conceptual plan was beginning to work.

About one-third of the way through the semester, the class focus shifted toward engagement with and at Luther Manor. Here, theory had to become practice. Basting and I became very practical—dealing with logistics, plans of action, instruction in person-centered care, group leadership, and group flow—shadowing our students as they made their initial visits. We rode the bus with students, modeled interactions, suggested alternative ideas, and encouraged reflection.

During site visits, faculty and students entered the Luther Manor Welcome Center together each week, greeted the receptionist Julianne, and donned our nametags. Then students dispersed into their four small groups throughout the care community—in the Terrace, Courtyards, Health Care Center, and Adult Day Center where Luther Manor program staff (as opposed to faculty) took on the direct oversight role. Basting and I would visit, observe, and document group sessions, but we did not intervene. We had built ambiguity into the conceptual framework of the project so that participation would not be limited to "correct answers" or routine outcomes. Groups were encouraged to develop creative end points, design freely, and focus on individual participants' insights and ideas. For example, one student group decided to invite its discussion group (in Luther Manor's Courtyards) to explore the meaning of "epics." In Greek society, everyone knew the story of Odysseus and Penelope. What is a story that everyone knows? That we can all participate in telling communally? Together their creative discussion group decided on the story of Cinderella. The students brought costumes for the elders to choose from as they retold the story for themselves.

While tremendous creativity flourished in this open format (as Basting and I had hoped), at this juncture students also confronted that inevitable experience most of us have when theoretical plans meet reality—cognitive dissonance. We began to sense both apprehension and even some mild fear. What was the right answer? What did success look like? How does one interact with people who are in wheelchairs or have oxygen tubes protruding from their noses? How could students tell if they were earning a "good grade"? All of these were legitimate questions. The need for clarity and clear boundaries was understandable and valid. Fear of failing, surprise when things went badly (or, for that matter, went well), and trepidation over meeting and connecting with people who were culturally and generationally divided from them created a good deal of anxiety.

There was no instruction manual for how to respond and interact. Basting and I had provided students with simulations and examples from pilot programs. We had used significant portions of the TimeSlips Creative Storytelling process, which teaches basic improvisational skills in health care settings. Still, this was new and unexplored territory for nearly all of the students. Add to this the fact that our students had formally reported (in pre-project surveys and questionnaires) that they were uncomfortable being around "old sick people," and we had a recipe for considerable curricular discomfort.

Our culture, in general, is youth-oriented. The elderly and infirm enter care facilities as they confront stressed resources and a need for expert medical care. Socially, however, this isolates seniors—especially as they become more disabled. We segregate elders in institutions or retirement communities, which are often built away from city centers. Our students are in a similar situation. In university settings, they are segregated by economics (they live in dorms or student ghettos) and socially (where interaction is heavily weighted toward youth-culture parties, media, and music and other events marketed toward the under-thirty crowd).

The Penelope courses required that students confront these societal norms and engage with a community that was, for the most part, outside of their daily familiar routine. So too for the elders at Luther Manor, who also had to adjust and respond to a wave of young adults arriving every Thursday afternoon. We discovered that this intergenerational encounter was an important step toward the success of the overarching Penelope Project. For Luther Manor residents, co-learning and creating with the students and artists was something to look forward to, a welcome change in routine:

> You think about how we look forward to going on a vacation. . . . What do a lot of our residents who are in the health care [area] have? There isn't anything. [Maybe they think], "I go down to lunch today — okay, maybe I am going down to the activity room and maybe I'm playing bingo today.". . . But this [project] was SOMETHING; I could see it as [the residents] come down, as they embraced the actors and the students. It was something to look forward to. (Luther Manor staff interview)

As the elders got used to the students, the students could sense their joy and appreciation of the students' efforts. This in turn deepened their engagement and increased the exploration of what was possible. It invited fresh perspectives from both students and elders alike. As one Luther Manor resident noted, "My overall experience was, 'Hooray for young people!' It felt good to be with young people again — no insult intended here — white hairs and all." Despite their trepidation, the students became excited and, at times, elated. They made important discoveries and connections. Speaking and interacting with elders had a powerful effect on students' values. We checked in at the end of each site visit by meeting back in the Welcome Center at Luther Manor. They excitedly and rapidly poured out stories, insights, and "Ah-Ha!" experiences.

Josh, for example, a UWM senior, arrived at one of these debriefing sessions in tears. He explained that he had just had a profound conversation with one of the members of his group — and it reminded him of his grandfather. Josh had then slipped away, called his grandfather using his cell phone, and had a conversation. Josh said, "I told him that I loved him — that I missed him. I don't visit him as much as I probably should." Other students had similar responses and told us that, before enrolling in the course, they thought their grandparents (or older aunts, uncles, etc.) were often silly or boring. Their work on Penelope radically changed this attitude.

Another stumbling block along the way was something that we refer to in education as "course-and-a-half syndrome." One tends to plan a new course by trying to put *everything* about the subject into it. The result is an overloaded system that encumbers the very progress one is trying to achieve. Clarity often takes repeated attempts to achieve. One student emphatically observed:

[These courses were] a pain, we were always too busy, we struggled to find time outside of our course work — which was almost impossible — I was busy from 7 am to 11 pm — BUT it was worth it. To see the faces of the folks at Luther Manor when we would work with them and how it made them feel to be around us — to be around young people like us. I would do it all over again.

It can be difficult to edit courses until one sees them in action. Teaching is an intuitive and constructed process just as much as it is a cerebral and cognitive one. It is only by doing the instruction that we get true insights into what we ought to have done, or might do next time. In our zealousness, we overplanned Penelope courses and created schema and materials that were too complicated. Our advice to others who want to try this type of work is to be a bit more practical at the start, simplify resources, and provide more time for explanation and reflection.

But, we were also lucky, or perhaps graced, that the resilience of our students emerged as their commitment to the project, and relationships within it, deepened. They were able to work through stress and focus on things they valued: exploring the *Odyssey*, engaging in intergenerational conversation, and connecting to each other. These aspects helped overcome the challenges and brought about transformation. This was evident in their end-of-semester team performances that they wrote and performed in front of over two hundred Luther Manor residents gathered in the Faith and Education Center. Inspired by their groups' discussions, these short plays incorporated bits of humor and personality from their groups' participants. They were funny, heartfelt, and well-executed. While these performances were not incorporated into the *Finding Penelope* production, the intergenerational bonding and excitement for creative exploration they created were integral to the overall success of the project and to the individual student success in the class. As one of the students noted:

The sheer size and scope of the project is just startling! And it is starting to hit me, that basic element, realizing what a huge thing we are doing! It's a huge thing and at the same time we are so comfortable together — with the residents at Luther Manor, I mean. I think that it's the comfort of it that is going to make it a success. This is WILD! It's BIG! It's TERRIFIC! And we do it together.

STUDENTS' EYE VIEW OF PENELOPE
Fly Steffens and Angela Fingard

FLY STEFFENS

I played the role of a student devising facilitator and assistant playwright. I was enrolled in both Storytelling and Playwriting II, with my playwriting project for the semester being to assist Dr. Anne Basting with drafts of *Finding Penelope*, the play to be staged by Sojourn Theatre.

The students in Storytelling were split up into small groups, each of which led sessions at Luther Manor. I was in the group working with the section of the Manor that functioned more as independent living than hospice or skilled care. I would have had a much different experience had I been placed in a different group. Before this project, I didn't have a relationship with aging or a relationship with dementia. I had both my grandparents at the time. I hadn't experienced any significant deaths or losses in my life as an adult, other than my own personal struggles with suicide and depression. But I had beaten that—and I was having a wonderful time being alive and intending on living an excellent, full, and long life with no consideration of how those around me or others might age or suffer from memory loss.

On one of the first days of Storytelling, prior to having even visited Luther Manor, we did an in-class exercise that asked us to envision ourselves in fifty to sixty years—as an "old person." We were asked to draw a picture, and I remember what I drew clearly: a woman with excessively long, flowing, gray, curly hair—covered shoulder to foot in tattoos, surrounded by stacks and stacks of books. Smiling.

And then we were asked how we pictured ourselves generally—and it became apparent that no one in the group had taken into consideration any disease they might encounter, any memory loss they might suffer, any fate that may take them sooner. I saw my piles of books fall away page by page and was faced with the idea of not being able to remember every story I've ever heard, every story I've ever told or will tell. The idea of looking down at my arms and not remembering why these pictures and words are embedded into my skin—knowing they are there but not knowing why. Or maybe not even knowing they are there.

So in the middle of the classroom chair circle, I started sobbing. Pretty uncontrollably. I'd already faced death in my life, but it was self-imposed and self-controlled in a way. Aging and the onset of memory loss would not be a thing over which I had much control, if any. It was facing death, physically and conceptually, in a way I had never considered. And thus I became the crier of the group—which is why I'm not sure how my participation in the project would have panned out had I been placed elsewhere. It's not that I was upset by or scared of those experiencing serious symptoms of dementia and other physical ailments in their old age—it was an overwhelming sense of empathy. There was a day you were me, and there may . . . there *will* be a day I am you—and now we are here together.

I think the experience at the beginning of the semester with drawing the picture of my "old self" lead me to take on more of an observer's role. I was treading unknown ground, for sure. I didn't realize that, even in my somewhat passive role as an observer, I was also being observed—the participants in our devising group at Luther Manor considered me to be thoughtful, quiet, and demure. Never before or since have I been described in this way, mind you, so I think I took a bit more of an active role at that point, especially when the group would describe characters in the *Odyssey* and their wants. The whiteboard picture we created together (they described; I drew) of Penelope is an image that will literally stay with me, in my mind and on my body, as a tattoo.

At the end of the semester, students were to take what we had transcribed and create a performance as a kind of celebration amongst the entire Manor. I played an elderly character, which seemed fitting—another student did my makeup on the bus; it was if I had come full circle from the beginning of the semester. I remember an intense feeling of sadness that this section of gathering stories and thoughts was over.

At this point my involvement shifted—I was involved in two other productions at the university as a writer/dramaturg/assistant director, so I was around for the really intense first devising week with Sojourn Theatre and then basically left until showtime.

Even though I spent a very short time with Sojourn Theatre, it was the first time I had seen their kind of process, and it influences me to this day—what devising means and how it changes depending on where you are or with whom you are working; what design means in a site-specific space; how the smallest things can constitute performance; how to make theatre accessible to a nontraditional audience or nontraditional performers. What I think of as being performative is wildly different now than it was before that process. I'm more open to experimentation—in fact, I crave it.

Through Penelope, I learned that not everyone will understand or remember what you're doing or what you've done, but it matters greatly that you do it. It matters to create meaningful engagement in the day-to-day lives of those living with dementia. It does make a difference. I've seen it. It is ephemeral, but it stays with you — in the core of you.

ANGELA FINGARD

In the fall of 2010, I returned to school to pursue a theatre degree as a mature student. I already had a master's degree in education, and I had worked in nonprofits doing community development and, later, in a large corporation doing organizational development. I chose theatre because I loved the idea of using the arts for teaching and community development. I knew nothing about the Penelope Project when I signed up for the Storytelling class with Anne Basting and Robin Mello, and when I learned about the project on my first day, I was blown away by the fortuitous timing of my return to school. I was a part of the Penelope Project for a full academic year.

During the first semester, we were asked to explore our feelings of aging and disease and learn about person-centered care. At the time, my grandmother had advanced Alzheimer's, and while I didn't live close to her, I felt very close to her and her caregivers. Despite this, I had not spent much time considering my own aging or the possibility of disease. By the end of this project I was brought closer to my grandmother, my future elderly parents, and my future elderly self in a way that is still indescribable.

I worked as a student devising facilitator with three other members of my class. We gathered stories from the Luther Manor residents who were living independently. While I felt quite comfortable with older people, I remember the feeling of anticipation every time we got on the bus to go to Luther Manor. I was so excited about the stories we'd hear, share, and be a part of creating, but I was also nervous about putting my foot in my mouth and saying something really naive, uncaring, or unfeeling. I had no idea what it was like to live an additional forty to fifty years on this planet, experience disease, lose physical ability, or lose very close loved ones. Within our student group, my role was to facilitate with the residents our thoughts from previous meetings and to guide the conversation through questions or themes we were exploring. The student team was very collaborative. We met often to recap what we were hearing and to discuss additional topics we wanted to cover. After a couple of meetings with both the students and the residents, the entire group felt like a safe, trusting environment, and everyone came very willing to share.

I'm sure it's possible that I and others might have stuck a foot in our mouths, but because of the incredible trust and love the group created, it became a safe, joyful space that allowed for real learning to occur.

From our discussion group in independent living, Luther Manor residents Rusty Tym and Joyce Heinrich wound up being actors in the Penelope play. Their energy, passion for life, and enthusiasm for the project helped build bridges between the students and the other residents. What I never knew until the end of the semester was how nervous they were about meeting us. Joyce wrote a very moving, insightful poem about her shift in attitude of spending time with us. She read the poem on our last day together, and it was an incredible gift. It felt like we'd come full circle; we all started in a place of uncertainty and insecurity and wound up feeling more deeply connected than we ever could have anticipated.

During the second semester, I was the assistant director of the Penelope play, working closely with Anne Basting, Maureen Towey, and Sojourn Theatre during the devising period and then again during rehearsals and performances. My role as assistant director included a lot of logistics, including coordinating with staff and volunteers about transporting Luther Manor residents with various physical abilities to the room for the final scene, the placement of each of the forty to fifty residents on stage for the final scene, and knowing their different ailments and interests so that I could position them in the place that would give them the most comfort. Then I would rehearse with all the residents who arrived. I was always filled with such anticipation, waiting for residents to arrive and not knowing how many would show up. Then slowly people would arrive, sometimes aided by walkers or canes and some in wheelchairs. We got such a great turnout that it was a question not of whether there would be enough people but, rather, of where would we put them all! The rehearsals were joyful and full of curiosity, confusion, questions, and concerns. Mainly they were filled with anticipation of being a part of something big. I would practice the call and response lines and then the gestures that went with the final poem. Once we got to the performance dates, I rehearsed with this impromptu chorus prior to every performance so that they felt ready and prepared. Some remembered from rehearsals, and those that didn't were shown where to look so that they knew whom to follow. The best way I can describe my role as assistant director in this project is as a really good host to a wonderful party. I needed to know my guests so well that I could anticipate their needs and any possible wants beforehand, then I would welcome them all and make them feel like the happy, honored guests that they were. Then I asked them to please join me in sharing words and gestures that created a very nourishing environment for all involved. Then I thanked them all profusely for coming and asked them to please come again and made sure they all got back comfortably and safely to their homes.

Expressing what I gained from this experience is challenging. Penelope is an all-encompassing feeling. The project had heart, a huge, pulsing heart that was pumping throughout Luther Manor and amongst every person directly or indirectly involved. The project was amazing throughout the process, during the play, and afterward. I witnessed a man, who had a stroke three years prior, engage fully in every rehearsal and performance. I heard from his wife afterward that he spoke his first full sentences since his stroke, explaining this project to his men's group, even demonstrating the choral gestures. I witnessed residents who had hidden talents that hadn't been revealed to fellow residents or staff until this project tapped into their creative side or until they were asked to help out. The huge hunger for this type of expression and inclusion from every member of this community created magic!

I learned new theatre skills like devising. I learned the joys and challenges of working within a health care system. I learned that there was no such thing as too much communication, especially since there were so many people involved with varying degrees of participation, responsibility, and concern for the safety of residents, buildings, or guests. A project of this scale requires a huge commitment from everyone involved in order for trust to build and lasting change to occur. But the most important thing I learned was the importance of feeling a part of a community, the importance of being a part of something bigger than yourself, to have a title or role separate from that of staff, caregiver, patient, or disease label.

My brother has a serious mental illness, and I often use communication techniques I learned from this project to engage with him. I occasionally work with people living with mental illness and love to create opportunities where they can shed their disease labels and be seen only as storytellers and artists. I will be forever grateful for all of those whom I encountered during the Penelope Project. My life is much richer for every single one of them.

ON THE COMFORT OF ENTERTAINMENT
Anne Basting

I have fond memories of going out to Luther Manor with my sister at Christmas time and strolling through the Day Center and singing to the participants. As Kirsten Jacobs observes in her essay in part one, this kind of entertainment is the dominant form of programming in long-term care. Let me play for you. Let me dance for you. Let me present a monologue for you. This kind of presentation is safe for both visitors and residents. It is the giving and receiving of a gift that makes both parties feel good. The entertainer doesn't really need to engage with or form relationships with the residents. The residents don't need to risk anything beyond clapping. Expectations are clear. Residents sit quietly, watch the visitor, and applaud (laugh, boo, etc.) at the appropriate time. And then the relationship is over. This type of exchange is orderly, which makes it easy for staff to schedule. The guitar player comes at ten. The children's choir comes at eleven. Then lunch.

Our goal from the start of the Penelope Project was to shift this model from entertainment toward creative collaboration—to create opportunities for residents, staff, families, students, and artists to create something together. Together, we thought, we would invite people to join our project as actors, designers, writers, and so forth. We made giant posters: We need actors! We need designers! Come join us!

No one came.

We underestimated the powerful desire and mechanisms for minimizing risk and maximizing efficiency in the long-term care setting, from both staff and residents. The lure of the entertainment model, to clap when appropriate, is that you don't need to say anything. Residents don't need to expose their disabilities, be they in hearing, speaking, memory, or some physical form. Staff can plan ahead (we've booked the guitar player for the third Tuesday of every month). Staff and residents alike were comforted by routine. By asking people to co-create, we were asking them to do something they couldn't plan. Even as we imagined we would grow people's abilities (even find some new ones), we were asking them to reveal their disabilities and leave their comfort zones.

No wonder no one came.

We adjusted by taking down the posters. We wouldn't ask people to DO or

BE anything, except come talk with us. We would grow together from there. Much like the mantra of the TimeSlips storytelling method ("There are no right answers! You can say anything! We're making it up together!"), we demonstrated that anyone could join us from wherever he or she was. Residents and families started to join the student-led creative discussion groups. Later, we invited two of those residents to play lead roles in the final theatre production itself.

As we transitioned from the creative discussions to the devising and staging of the play, the lure of the entertainment model never went away. After a weeklong visit by Sojourn in October 2010, we felt a spike in the excitement and interest level. Luther Manor staff confirmed this. "Everyone wants to be a part of it now," said Beth Meyer-Arnold at our exit meeting for that week. In response, when I wrote the first draft of the play, I created a "chorus" that would play Penelope in the end and speak simple, echoed lines throughout the play itself. Whenever anyone heard the word "Penelope," he or she would say, "Our cunning, noble, wise, and loving queen," even if the person were just passing by in the hallway and not actually in the scene.

But when we introduced the idea of a chorus to residents in January during our first devising week, it met a familiar wall of resistance. A chorus? I can't sing. I can't memorize. I can't commit to being there for every performance. I want to watch the performance, not be in it. Staff explained that residents were too worried to join the chorus. In one meeting, nearly two weeks from the first performances, this issue came to a head in one of our regular staff/artist meetings. I remember someone asking, "How will we get all the residents in the Terrace to see the play if there are only fifty tickets per show?" I said, "If everyone in the Terrace sees the show instead of being in it, this project has failed."

Now that's not totally fair. There were really cool things happening all over the care campus with this show. Two performers had a choreographed snowball fight outside one of the windows. Jackie (a resident) played "Sentimental Journey" on the keyboard in a magical moment of blurring—is this normal life in the care center? Or is this the play? There was a sword fight in the Courtyards dining room. Someone crawled through a window (in a care center!) in scene 1. People wanted to see it. I wanted to see it too. They wanted to support their friends Rusty and Joyce in their professional acting debuts. We had been unable to include the Terrace (independent senior apartments) in the journey of the play because it was just too far for people to walk, so they wouldn't get to see a scene staged in their own area as the Health Care Center and the Courtyards would.

To find a middle ground, we created several preview performances that would enable people to see it *and* be in it. Slowly, from preview rehearsals through the performances themselves, the number of people in the chorus grew. In the opening scene, the chorus began with three people reading right from copied scripts. By the final show, I was madly copying scripts. There were twenty-five to thirty people jammed into the spot behind the doors where the chorus shouted their lines, from the silly to the sublime. Some chorus members followed the audience to the Health Care Center and Welcome Center to watch the first two scenes, then came back down to play Penelope in the final chorus. "Penelope to places in the Faith and Education Center. Penelope to places," called the announcer over the campus-wide public address system.

We found a way to reduce the fears of memorization and commitment as well. We simply said, "Come if you can." We had no sign-up sheets. No solid numbers of how many people we needed. No scripts. Sojourn performer Nikki Zaleski sat in front of the chorus, and the chorus would echo her words and movements. It was terrifying for us as artists. This was our big finale. What if when Odysseus opened the curtains to reveal his cunning, noble, wise, and lovely queen — no one had shown up that day? But by letting go of expectations, we made it possible for people to join us. The final chorus also grew during the performances. We started with maybe a dozen. And by the final performance, there were forty people on stage. Family members. Staff. Residents in hospice. Residents in independent living. There was an audible gasp during the shows when Odysseus would peek through the curtain. Both sides were surprised and excited that the other had shown up. "Welcome home Odysseus," the chorus of Penelope relayed through the "Welcome Dance" that Luther Manor residents themselves had written and created: "Our hearts are open to you. Our soul and our spirit welcome you home. I am calling you. I am hearing you. I am seeing you. Your eyes sparkle like the stars." Together, we had created home and were welcoming the audience — to Luther Manor, to ancient Greece, to the magic of what co-creation makes possible.

THE FIRST REHEARSAL
Maureen Towey

As the director of *Finding Penelope*, I remember entering the nursing wing for our first rehearsal and feeling terrified. We had been through the nursing wing before, and I braced myself every time, preparing for a room full of people in wheelchairs with a wide mix of physical and mental capacities, people who have been categorized as the most ill in the community. Jeanne, the extraordinary activity staff person in this area, has already arranged the room and helped to position everyone's wheelchairs so they are ready to collaborate with us. The professional cast and I huddle to the side for a few minutes, chatting nervously amongst ourselves — clearly delaying because we do not know how to start.

For a long moment, I look around and think that I have made a grave mistake by asking esteemed artists to collaborate with this marginalized and unpredictable population. *I can't do it. We have to postpone. We have to find another way to do this.* Sensing this internal panic, Anne reminds me that all I need to do to begin is to greet people. The entire room is looking toward me to lead, so I shake off my doubts, kneel down, and introduce myself to a woman in a wheelchair.

The goals of my theatre rehearsals are discovery, embodiment, repetition, and refinement. I have faith that the residents have the power of discovery, and we are slowly learning that they can embody ideas within a certain framework. But, knowing that most of these residents have profound memory issues, I wonder, will they be able to repeat anything that we discover today?

Before we can even deal with issues of memory, we have a more immediate problem — most of the residents have trouble hearing, and some of them don't see very well either. I have to turn the volume way up on my style of directing — each directive is given slowly and loudly, my gestures are emphatic, and my collaborators are throughout the room, echoing me and attending to residents who may have a hard time seeing me.

I tell everyone about the scene that we're going to work on: Penelope will be endlessly weeping behind closed doors, and they will be her chorus, supporting their queen and lamenting her troubles. We read through the scene. Normally in these moments I would be attending closely to my lead actors, helping with staging and clarity, but I can't do that while maintaining the momentum of the entire group. We will have to work out the nuance of the scene later. For now, the main task is to get the room to weep alongside their queen. I ask the group, how might you show someone crying? One woman slowly pulls her fingers down her face. I repeat this simple weeping gesture to the rest of the group. We model the gesture, and the residents mirror back what they see. Anne asks, "What would it sound like?" And they respond with a low, moaning crying sound.

We try it out at three different levels of sound and movement. Can you try the crying again? This time make it BIG? This time LITTLE? This time MEDIUM? It's a simple rehearsal strategy, but here, with the sounds of crying going from a whimper to a hyperbolic full-on sob, it feels profound. Their hand gestures grow and shrink with the volume of the tears. The group is laughing—and pretend-crying. There is freedom in putting on a mask of despair—especially in this room, where despair was what we were afraid of encountering. They are getting the hang of what it means to rehearse. We repeat the scene over and over again so that people can practice. This part feels like a normal rehearsal—you discover what works; you repeat and refine.

At one point, as we are working on the crying gesture, I kneel down to work individually with a resident named Elizabeth. Her frail body sits in a high-backed, wheeled recliner chair. Her head hangs low into her chest, her torso unable to sit up, though her gaze and voice are direct and clear. She says to me, "Sometimes it is good to cry." I can't quite believe what I'm hearing so I lean in closer; she holds my hand and says it again, "Sometimes it is good to cry," and she is actually crying a little bit. For a moment, I wonder if I have upset her, if the work we are doing is damaging in some way, but there is something in this moment that I recognize from other rehearsals I've been in. Elizabeth is connecting to the material in a visceral way. As she is crying, I can see her giving me a small smile.

At the end of rehearsal, I am exhausted, and Elizabeth grabs my hand again and tells me I did a good job. I feel so relieved and gratified to hear her say that.

We all finish rehearsal feeling a little bit triumphant. But will our newly rehearsed chorus remember anything of what we have built? The next day on a break, I go to visit Elizabeth, convinced I have found a replacement grandmother during my time in Milwaukee. I lean in close, as we did the day before, but she does not know who I am.

Right.

Of course. Working with people living with dementia can be filled with little heartbreaks. The memory issues of the group posed challenges, but, in truth, forgetfulness became valuable and forgiving. If I staged the scene poorly the first time, I could entirely change it the next time and no one would complain. There were no expectations of failure. Instead, I had total freedom to imagine a scene anew with each rehearsal.

We return for rehearsals day after day, and, to maintain consistency, at every rehearsal we practice our crying gestures. To my surprise, about three weeks in, our chorus in the nursing wing starts to improve. They anticipate their cues, their timing becomes more acute, and they are clearly enjoying themselves, which is often the key to a great performance. It felt as if we were reinventing what it means to remember.

When it came time for performances, the chorus in the nursing wing was always one of the highlights of the play. In fact, some of our performers became comfortable enough that they would improvise. At our final performance, Nancy, a resident with a mischievous streak, was supposed to be sitting with some weaving in her lap and watching the main actors in the scene. But slowly and with great effort, she started to lift the weaving from her lap until she was holding it over her head, stealing the spotlight for a moment, her face beaming, and looking as if she had just won something.

THE DEMANDS OF A PAINTER, OR WHO IS AN ARTIST?

Ellie Rose

Penelope invited all Luther Manor community members, residents, staff, and volunteers to contribute and engage in the project, even those outside of our walls. The life enrichment specialists and nurses were the key staff responsible for the implementation of Penelope. Administrators were included because their buy-in was crucial to enabling activity structures to change and the project's success to be valued. Looking back, I see now that we overlooked some departments because we assumed they were not directly working with residents. This is a story of how Penelope inspired me to expand my perceptions of the people that compose the Luther Manor community.

There are only two painters for Luther Manor's twenty-two-acre building, out of more than fifteen people on Luther Manor's maintenance team. There are approximately 740 resident rooms, sixteen dining rooms, twenty large programming spaces (plus multitudes of smaller spaces), and miles and miles of hallways. Into this maintenance system, I put my work order in for the ceiling of A206 to be painted a sky-blue using two cans of used house paint. A206 would now be known as "Penelope's Room" and act as a gallery for all our creative output.

What is a work order? It is a half-sheet, carbon-copy form composed of date, department, supervisor, and description requests. I filled out the work order and forced myself to be as concrete and direct as possible, omitting artsy words like "abstract," "expressive," and "whimsical." A maintenance team certainly wouldn't appreciate my attempts to flood Penelope's Room with the arts and creativity.

Then I met Lori.

I went to Penelope's Room to see if the ceiling had been completed so I could invite a small group to start sketching our Greek landscape mural on the wall. When I walked in the door, I was welcomed with a stressed hello and a rushed "I'm almost done, I will be right out!" I looked up and saw a beautiful blue sky with abstracted, expressive, whimsical clouds. I was speechless. I continued to watch as Lori stretched her arms, sponging in cloud forms and then adding expressive strokes of blue to work back into the abstract sky. I expressed my amazement over and over again, but none of the words seemed to fit the gratitude I was trying to convey. I told her she didn't have to do what she did (this was a lot of extra work), but she humbly responded that it was not an inconvenience. She continued to express that she had to mix the two cans to get the color she did and that she was happy to put in the extra time for something that would be enjoyed by so many residents.

I decided to leave the artist to finish, and as I was going out the door she asked me to leave the door open so residents could come in and say hello. When I returned, she informed me of the empty nail holes she filled and gave me instructions about how to fill the ones she had missed. She turned to her painting cart and said, "A present for you . . . extra hole filler just in case." I laughed because it was her heart that would be the present for all who entered Penelope's Room. As she added her final artistic touches, she openly shared the demands of being a painter in Luther Manor. We silently gazed together at the beauty she created, and I whispered, "Masterpiece."

As I left the room I was kicking myself for being so naive and judgmental. Why had I not invited one of our talented painters to be a part of this project? Why did I look at it as a "work order" and not as a personal contribution? I learned a great lesson from Lori on Friday. Penelope (and her room) brings together the many, many people who make up Luther Manor. She consistently shows us that anyone can be abstract, expressive, and even whimsical. We just need to invite and welcome them.

OPEN AND ROVING REHEARSALS
Michael Rohd and Maureen Towey

Theatre rehearsals generally happen in a closed studio environment. This was not the case for *Finding Penelope*. The show was site-specific — it was created in and for a specific location. The play itself was a journey during which an audience moved through a long-term care facility. This meant that to rehearse the show, we had to work in that facility. The performance space was an active, living environment, so every rehearsal became not only a testing ground for artistic ideas but also an opportunity for building community around the project and goodwill for the event. Essentially, by moving through Luther Manor with us, audience members became characters in the play and in the lives of hundreds of residents and staff members. We plotted the staging with great care. So, while having an open rehearsal can sometimes be a daunting, vulnerable situation, it was necessary for us because it kept us deeply entwined into the daily rhythms of Luther Manor.

When we were first getting to know the buildings of Luther Manor, we spent many hours wandering the hallways. We searched for spaces that would be great for performance and where it would also be possible to host daily rehearsals. For example, the lobby was a place that people passed through, but nobody really owned it, so our rehearsal work there would not be too disruptive. The lobby also provided us with a lovely sliding window — while it was usually used for food service, we used it as a puppet stage, allowing our performance to start with a moment of surprise and transformation. While working in the lobby area, we made sure to leave clear pathways so that residents could pass through or stop in as we worked. We hoped that our artistic conversations would soon seem as regular as any other conversation in the common spaces of Luther Manor. We hoped that, eventually, Luther Manor would feel like a place where art was being made — anywhere, at any time.

Although the lobby was a natural choice for rehearsals, the dining hall was not. We were drawn to its wide windows and location at the heart of the assisted living wing called the Courtyards. Some staff discouraged our initial interest because the dining hall patterns of activity were ingrained and inflexible. Delaying the staff efforts there would cost money. Many of the residents in the Courtyards depended on the regularity of the meal schedule to structure their days and give them a sense of clarity. So, when we started to play in the space, there was confusion from some residents. They would start to line up on the benches outside the dining hall an hour before meals, and we would be staging an epic battle scene or improvising a new dance. We had to enlist staff to be rehearsal assistants for the residents — sometimes they were able to engage residents in our work; sometimes it was easier to steer their focus elsewhere. The dining hall ended up being our most successful performance space, but the rehearsals required daily assessment and negotiation with the staff members who, at times, perceived our work as making their jobs more difficult.

Open rehearsals enabled us to prove our commitment to the project to staff. If staff felt at all as if we were behaving like highfalutin artists, seeing ourselves as removed from their daily lives, we would break the trust we'd built up so carefully. We had to be inviting staff, families, volunteers, and residents to engage with the project at every step. There were seven hundred people on staff, so the process of communication had to be ongoing. There was no way we were going to reach all seven hundred people at once. It was a day-to-day process. That meant respectfully engaging with the dining hall workers, striking up conversations with the janitors, and looking for unexpected allies around every corner.

For the artists and actors reading this, many will be unsettled. It is difficult to make rich and complicated artistic decisions without some degree of control over your rehearsal environment. This way of working takes considerable flexibility and openness from the performers. The Sojourn actors are also, uniquely, very comfortable as facilitators. They knew their behavior on rehearsal breaks was as important as their work in the scenes. And, of course, we did find time to cocoon a little bit and figure out the more complicated performance choices. That type of work is essential in keeping the aesthetic qualities of the performance high.

For instance, in the final scene, performer James Hart had a lengthy monologue with the chorus. He really hit it out of the park in performance even though there wasn't a lot of time to prepare him in terms of moment-to-moment work. The chorus was in flux each day so we didn't know how many people would be onstage and how exactly James would be able to negotiate that crowd. James was so open to input and interaction, but, as the script was changing, there were days when he basically said, "I need time to step away, memorize this, and quietly figure out what I'm doing with this scene." For our performers to do their best work, making room for that attention to detail was essential.

We found balancing inclusion and rigor to be an interesting parallel to the daily work of staff members who work at these long-term care communities. They are dealing with constant requests for their time and attention. How do they find the time to do their jobs as well as they would like and still stay engaged? We were very impressed with the Luther Manor staff, in terms of how adaptive they were within their own work lives while maintaining a high standard of work.

We also found interesting parallels between the type of privacy that you relinquish in an open rehearsal environment and the way privacy can be compromised in a care setting. The artists need quiet time to work, but they also need the support and input of the community to make a robust performance. Many residents enter Luther Manor because they need the care and supervision of a trained staff, but they also value their autonomy. In both the artistic and the care settings, we are trying to negotiate the role of the individual in an environment that is necessarily collaborative.

While open rehearsals took a great deal of persistence and negotiation, we believe they paid off in the end, particularly in the spaces where we had the least amount of control: the hallways. There are miles and miles of hallways at Luther Manor. For us, they became long, skinny performance spaces, but they also contain hundreds of literal doors into people's homes. At each rehearsal, as we transitioned between spaces, we would quietly parade through the hallways, greeting residents as we walked. So, when it came time to open up the performances to the public, these greetings naturally remained.

When audiences entered the first hallway of Luther Manor, residents opened their doors and waved. Most of these residents were in wheelchairs. It was an incredibly inclusive moment, but, also, in an artistic frame it embodied what we want from an actor onstage — an intimacy that is both effortless and complicated. When those residents opened their doors, they were saying, "This is my home, this is my room, this is my disability, and I am welcoming you." They came through the piece for maybe thirty seconds, and many of them we knew only because we were friendly as we passed their doors every day — but their participation was potent and memorable. This may have been one of the greatest things we learned from this process: when working in a community-engaged, site-specific process, the frame is everything. Giving residents the right frame gives them the same power, in their own homes, as a great actor on the stage. Each is choosing, in their moment of being seen, what to share and how to share it. That takes an openness on the part of all the collaborators. That openness is what the open rehearsal process allowed us to find.

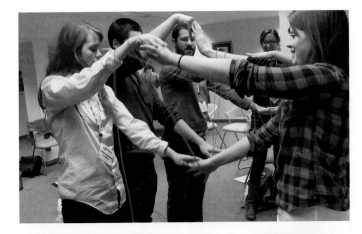

Sojourn rehearses. Nikki Zaleski, James Hart, Maureen Towey, Maggie McGwin. Photograph by Anne Basting.

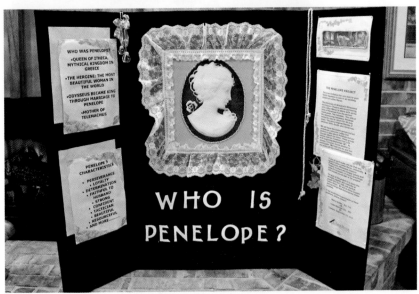

"Who Is Penelope?" display in Luther Manor's Terrace. Photograph by Anne Basting.

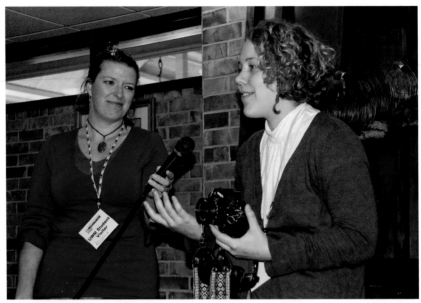

uwm students
Angela Fingard and
Fly Steffens facilitate
a discussion about
Penelope at Luther
Manor's Terrace.
Photograph by Anne
Basting.

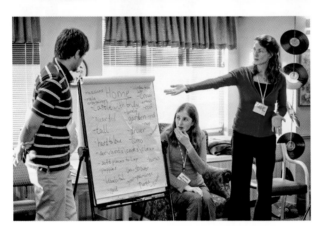

uwm students Rohit Ratagaran and Kathryn Otten facilitate
a poem about the meaning of "home" with Anne Basting.
Photograph by uwm Photo Services.

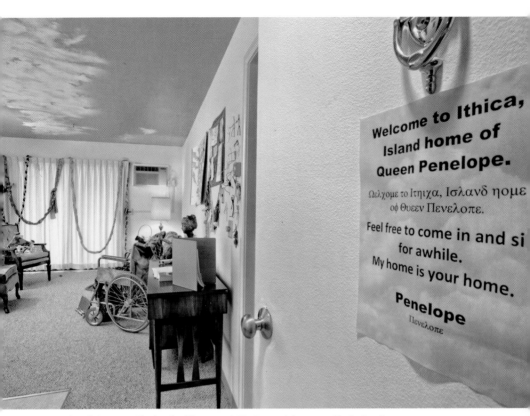

Penelope's Room, with cloud ceiling panel. Photograph by UWM Photo Services.

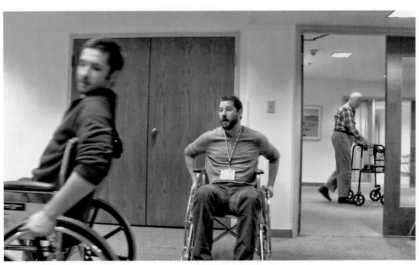

Sojourn's Daniel Cohen and James Hart in open rehearsals where residents are invited to stop in to share in the creative discovery.

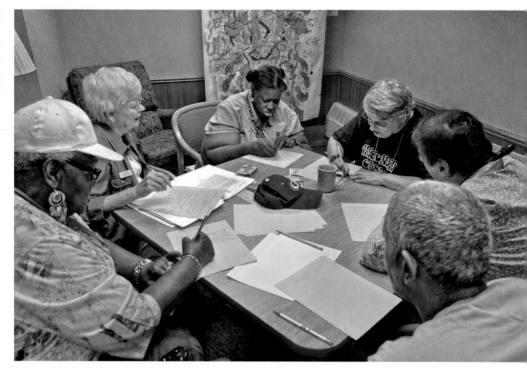

Luther Manor volunteer Jolene Hansen leads a letter-writing session with participants in Luther Manor's Adult Day Center. What would Penelope write to Odysseus? Photograph by UWM Photo Services.

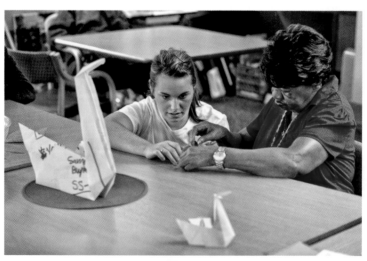

A student facilitates origami folding activity at Luther Manor's Adult Day Center. Photograph by UWM Photo Services.

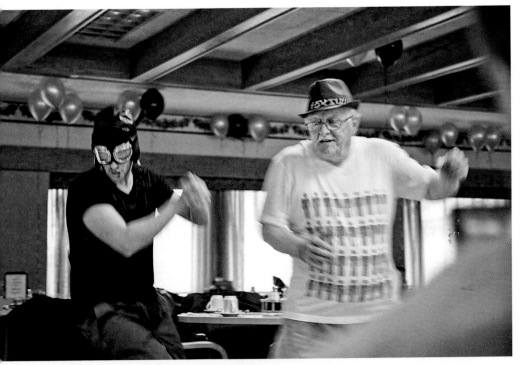

Daniel Cohen and Rusty Tym portray 108 suitors in *Finding Penelope*.
Photograph by UWM Photo Services.

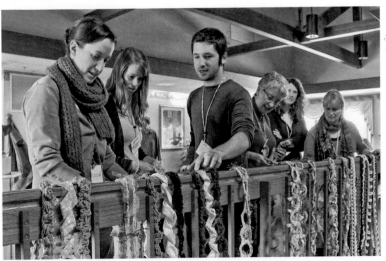

Sojourn performers and Luther Manor staff marvel at pieces of the three-quarter-mile-long weaving by residents that would eventually mark the path that the play *Finding Penelope* would take through Luther Manor. Photograph by 371 Productions.

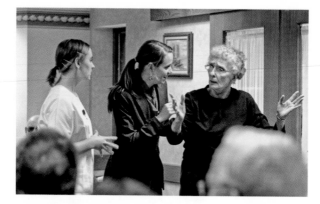

UWM student Julia Huryk, Sojourn's Nikki Zaleski, and Luther Manor's Joyce Heinrich entice "Penelope" to come out of her chamber—but she won't stop crying. Photograph by UWM Photo Services.

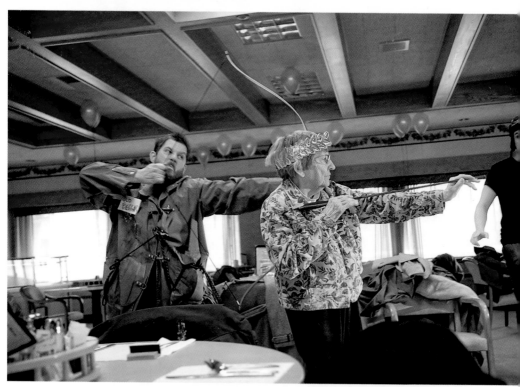

Sojourn's James Hart plays Odysseus and Luther Manor's Caroline Imhoff is Athena. Together they shoot an arrow through twelve axe handles in a test to win Penelope's love. Photograph by UWM Photo Services.

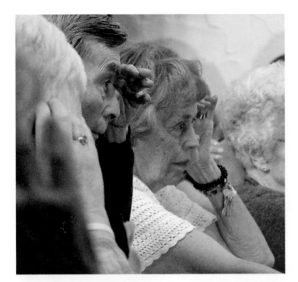

A chorus of Luther Manor residents portrays Penelope in the final scene of *Finding Penelope*. Photograph by 371 Productions.

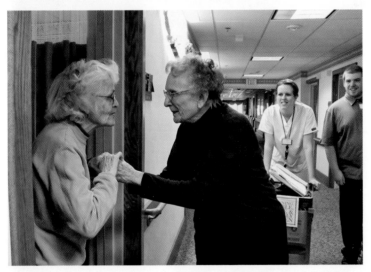

Luther Manor's Joyce Heinrich greets friend Lois Finger along the path of the *Finding Penelope* performance. Photograph by 371 Productions.

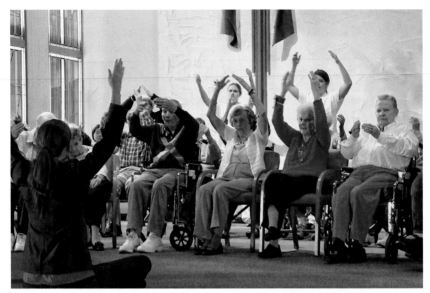

"Penelope," played by a chorus of residents, follows Sojourn's Nikki Zaleski through a series of movements and words. No memorization was necessary, making it possible for everyone to participate. Photograph by 371 Productions.

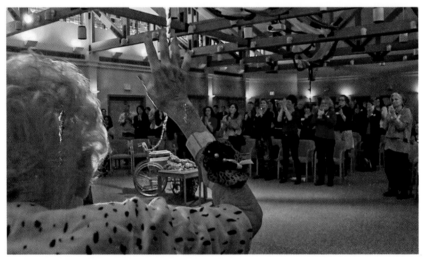

The audience for *Finding Penelope* as seen from the stage and the chorus playing Penelope. Photograph by 371 Productions.

PART FOUR: *Rewards*

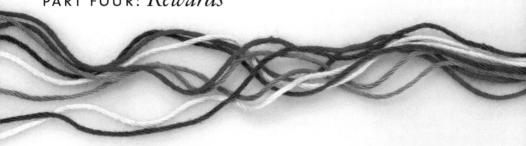

These relationships were not a sidebar to the project itself—they were core to the success of Penelope.
—Nikki Zaleski, Sojourn Performer

In part three, we focused on challenges and the adjustments we made in response to them. In part four, we look at the shining moments that emerged from those challenges and at those moments when we simply got the hang of Penelope—of how to invite each other to create together and what that could mean for the full community. These rewards included the impossibly long weaving crafted by hundreds of hands; the positive shifts in personal relationships; the power of gesture and story-telling; and the intergenerational friendships that bloomed and matured. This section details the circuitous routes and risks we took to find connection, clarity, and beauty. Once again, this section presents the project from multiple perspectives—artists, staff, volunteers, and residents. Shannon Scrofano (Sojourn Theatre's designer) and Ellie Rose of Luther Manor open the section with an overview of the breadth of art-making projects embedded in Penelope. They are followed by Luther Manor volunteer Jolene Hansen's poems crafted in collaboration with Luther Manor's Day Center participants. A series of dialogue essays follow—capturing the intergenerational friendships that grew from the project, in spite of a mountain of self-doubt and apprehension. Finally, Anne Basting and dancer/choreographer Leonard Cruz share the story of discovering the movement for the project, and Maureen Towey tells of the unique challenges of wrapping up an emotional two-year-plus project all in the final scene of a play.

THE ARTS OF PENELOPE:
ART-MAKING AND MAKING ARTIFACTS
Ellie Rose and Shannon Scrofano

Engaging in the arts within a long-term care community meant we had to first acknowledge the appreciation, safety, and comfort of existing arts and crafts programming. Activity calendars in long-term care settings across the country most commonly reflect the intent to support the human potential to express one's self creatively by offering traditional activities that physically create products such as glazed ceramic figurines and independently designed table centerpieces. These products promote self-worth, social confidence, and engagement — foundational values of Luther Manor's philosophy of person-centered care.

Before Penelope, Luther Manor had a rich history of executing engaging, art-based programs, specifically through our partnership with UWM faculty and students. We had a well-established schedule for storytelling, painting classes, music appreciation, and dance exercise. Yet, similar to our arts and crafts programs, the interests and interactions within these programs was becoming static and routine. Art-making was seen as being only for artists and those interested in becoming one.

Penelope's art-making dared to cross the boundaries of arts and crafts to include vision, intent, and the actual ideas of the community members involved. Elders, staff members, and volunteers became conscientious generators of their own creative processes. In the process, residents became empowered, staff members grew inspired, volunteers grew in number, and residents began to direct their own activities. The words, humor, stories, and creative abilities of the Luther Manor community ignited culture change by teaching and influencing the strangers outside and within our walls to value, respect, and build relationships as a necessity for personal and organizational growth.

As a visual artist and person-centered care specialist staff member at Luther Manor, Ellie Rose's role was translating the culture of Luther Manor to the project's partners, modeling engagement strategies, and executing the visual arts elements. As lead project designer, Shannon Scrofano's role was to develop and examine the asset map of Luther Manor and to uncover the quirks and details of locations that could be illuminated, enhanced, or subverted as a part of the performance's journey through the buildings. Our leadership and reflections supported the engagement and products of Penelope, and this artful exchange harvested many experiences for our personal growth as community artists. We share these lessons through dialogue in the hopes of inviting more voices to explore and attest to the power of art-making in a community. After the brief dialogue, we share short descriptions of several specific art-making invitations.

What did we learn about art-making within an existing community?
Shannon: Perhaps the answer to this question begins with the sources of creative activity. Broadly, creative acts — whether art, craft, or tinkering — may emerge out of curiosity, out of compulsion (to express, to articulate, to interrogate, to overthrow), or even out of boredom. Sometimes acts respond to need — identified by the maker themselves or identified by someone else. This is often cast as an act of design. As an educator, and as a designer working in community contexts, I ruminate frequently on art-by-invitation. In a classroom, that may be the response to an assignment or to an instruction; in communities, the creative response to a question or an open opportunity to participate in some way. At Luther Manor, I walked into a terror of possibilities — existing structures and classes that were largely organized by medium, yet provided frameworks for facilitating other creative invitations.

   Do acts by external invitation produce different results than when someone engages in a creative act of their own accord? In the best scenario, I think they can result in a kind of citizenship. That's how the idea of Penelope's weaving came about in working with Ellie at Luther Manor. The large weaving endeavor would create a structure that people could put themselves into. Like a sprawling welcome carpet running through over a half mile of hallways, made by the hands of the people who lived, worked, volunteered, and visited there, humbly aspiring to Robert Irwin's conception of folk art as an infusion of your personality and feelings into everyday objects. One segment of weaving by itself is a craft project, but, in great quantities, it becomes something else, bigger than the sum of its parts — its own independent invitation, a continuous guide along the journey of the play, evidence of invested hands.

Ellie: Just as Shannon described, art-making within an existing community "invites" members to embark on adventure. It inspires continuous learning and exploration of the unknown. It ignites curiosity, expands possibility, and embraces what it means to be present. These are universal and ageless desires. They don't stop at the doors of a nursing home. My person-centered experience has always supported me in making art with older adults because it challenges me to always recognize and rely on the abilities of the individuals. I am both intrigued and excited to learn about the emotions, life experiences, interests, and cognitive processes of elders because they are each unique. I learned that replacing expectation with invitations to contribute to a communal goal opened endless doors of creative possibility. With the support of the Penelope Project's partners, the Luther Manor community became fearless creators.

What was the significance of the weaving?

Shannon: The weaving, for me, collided useful imagery in the performance journey. In the myth of Penelope, the weaving is a means of waiting. It binds acute patience, waiting for the return of Odysseus from twenty years of war, with active resistance — a gutsy act of defiance in staving off suitors, freeloaders, and the cultural expectation that she is obligated to remarry. It also looked like all the images I was studying of tau protein models in individuals with dementia. The neurofibrillary "tangles" — dense tumble-weeds of dead or dying fragments and nerve cells — clustered around brain cells. They are considered insoluble.

    The idea of a single sculptural event that demonstrated a spectrum of participation felt so right for this project — from the professional, intricate, loomed acts of weaving or elaborate knitting capacity of some of the volunteers and independent living residents to the deeply expressionistic or circumstantial creations of participating weavers who may not recognize their own work only moments later, but instead see the possibilities for what is still to do. Like Penelope's, Luther Manor's weaving expresses waiting, choice, and resistance. Hung through a half mile of hallways, dining rooms, and common spaces, the audience, weavers, and performers are all engaged in the act of being "with" the weaving. It navigates the ways our brains work, remember, start anew, loop, struggle back — the way our brains may change in the future, toward creation of new images.

Ellie: The weaving is such a strong symbol of the power of the arts because it holds the functional and historical properties of an artifact, and the process of it coming into existence — art-making — has allowed it to radiate a communal energy. At first, it was installed in a jagged, horizontal line that continued down hallways, up walls, across nursing stations, avoiding fire sprinkler heads (by eighteen inches to be exact), and down stairwells. Its function was to mark the route of the play, and every moment that passed (even to this day) adds to its historical value of those from the artists of the past who made it.

After the *Finding Penelope* performance, the weaving was reinstalled in vertical, draping groups to lure viewers to walk through the weaving, to feel and touch it, just as the artists did when creating it. From there, pieces of it were given to family members to remember their loved one's contribution, and the rest was composed, piece-by-piece, paralleling one another and hung down a wall in the Day Center gallery. Strangers continued to come into our home, and Penelope's weaving welcomed them. They would pass through on their way to other care areas and rave about its beauty. Residents would talk about their contributions, and staff members would stop and tell their own stories of Penelope. The weaving was a celebration of what it means to wait and what we can create when we do.

Weaving

Artists: Hundreds of Luther Manor residents, staff, and volunteers

Media: Numerous small-group gatherings repeating patterns while exchanging stories, independent undertakings of crochet and knitting skill mastering, donated and discarded fibers (fabric, ribbons, yarn, etc.), and plastic six-pack rings

Communal Goal: Create a visual element to provide directions for the route of the play; transform a skilled-nursing dining room by adding elements of art — color, line, shape, form, texture, etc. — to the existing architecture of the dining spaces, living rooms, Welcome Center, and hallways

Love Letters to Penelope

Artists: Adult Day Center and Health Care Center participants and volunteer Jolene Hansen

Media: Share ideas about what Penelope may have felt waiting for her beloved husband for twenty years, poetry practice, pens, paper, scribe, word processor

Communal Goal: Write a love letter to Odysseus from Penelope

Origami Birds

Artists: Adult Day Center and Health Care Center participants and staff person

Media: Staff person fascination with origami, problem-solving exhibition options for the Love Letters to Penelope, the actual love letters

Communal Goal: Transform the love letters into a form that would help them get to Odysseus

Penelope's Room

Artists: Multiple staff persons, residents, and volunteers

Media: Greek city mural, ceiling sky mural, paint, bookshelf, writing desk, display wall, weaving room, seating, storage, signage

Communal Goal: Personalize a gathering place for individuals from all care areas in a vacant independent living apartment

Things We Don't Like / Things We Endure

Artists: Penelope room visitors

Media: Wax sticks, exhibit wall, small-group discussion of things we do not like

Communal Goal: Create dimensional visual forms of things in life people are "enduring" ("remain under," in ancient Greek) or do not like as a metaphor for the many suitors pursuing Penelope in order to become the next king of Ithaca

Home

Artists: Participating viewers and actors of *Finding Penelope*

Media: Acoustic rendition of the song "Home," originally written and recorded by Edward Sharpe and the Magnetic Zeros; electric piano version of "Sentimental Journey"

Communal Goal: Repeat a song while walking to the next scene location in the play to build excitement and set context for the final scene; in the opening scene, a resident musician, living with low vision, exhibits her piano expertise and creates a blur between the performance and the "real life" of Luther Manor

Welcome Dance

Artists: Choral actors in *Finding Penelope*

Media: Choreographer and dancer Leonard Cruz's teaching of Hawaiian
Gestural Dance to residents and participants across Luther Manor
Communal Goal: To create a "Welcome Dance" that serves to welcome
Odysseus home after his twenty-year absence and, in effect, welcome the
audience to Luther Manor

Penelope's Tea
Artists: Health Care Center residents, staff, and actors
Media: Tea, castle cake
Communal Goal: Gather to exchange ideas and celebrate Penelope

Cookie Mountain
Artists: Residents and actors
Media: Lots of cookies, glue, frosting
Communal Goal: Play with and exaggerate the symbol of the cookie and
how it is used to welcome strangers into homes

WHO IS A HERO IN YOUR OWN LIFE?

Jolene Hansen

One topic that arose in the Penelope discussions was "heroes." As a volunteer, I had time to talk with participants in the Day Center, one-on-one, about ordinary heroes in their lives. I look back on these personal encounters as gifts from Penelope. I was able to use the hero concept to enter into meaningful, everyday conversations — another example of what was happening "in the quiet corners" of the Penelope Project. In a journal I kept during the project, these encounters took on a poem-like form.

BERTHA

With catchy smile, ready eyes
she searches for words
heroes, yes, oh heroes
mother, father worked hard
in the house, barn, in the yard
my hero was Dolly
our horse of dapple gray
we loved her   she knew we did
we'd lay on her belly, hug her
"Dolly does more for us
than we do for her," Dad said
we cried when Dolly died
oh, how we cried

I'm relaxed now,
thinking of Dolly
Tears come a sigh a slow smile.

MARY

Sits with purpose, strong
though legs are weak
eyes flutter closed but mind tracks
with sure voice she speaks
words molded, profound

I was raised to do for myself.
I try to be sweet. Sometimes
the devil gets in there, like arthritis.
Mother taught me, "If you don't feel well,
keep a smile on your face."
Her eyes close she smiles.

ESTHER

Sits straight, pert
walker close by
black hat trimmed in red
perched just right
to catch the tilt of her head
as she listens, engages
with edgy comments
wise retorts.
Patience is a virtue,
she quotes her mother
who managed nine children.
I'm the youngest,
just my sister and me left.

Words come easily lately,
she reveals.
Someone is listening.

MARLENE

Sits hunched in her wheel chair
jacket over sweater over shirt
over meager bones.
With gravelly voice,
she sighs with resignation
her tool to cope with slow-passing days.
Just waiting to die.
The bitter edge of her voice pushes against hope.
A question softens the corners of her mouth
her voice warms, her mind sharpens.
Someone is listening.

MAMIE'S STORY
Beth Meyer-Arnold

It was a sunny, bright early November day as I walked from my office in the Day Center to my aunt Marion's room. I call her Aunt Mamie. She lives at Luther Manor, in the Health Care Center area. I had been on vacation and at a conference the few days before, so I didn't know how she would be when I saw her after being gone for ten days.

As I rounded the corner, she was at the mirror, trying to comb her hair with her nondominant hand, because of a recent rotator cuff tear. Her expression was of complete frustration, disappointment, and defeat—a woman, trying to look her best, put lipstick and powder on and touched up her hair; now all these daily tasks have become mountains. When she saw me, she dropped her hand with the comb in it and sighed. "Oh, Beth. I am so glad you are here."

We talked. I rattled on about the conference, how interesting it was, all the important people from my field coming together in Milwaukee to discuss the future of adult day services. Then our lovely, warm vacation in southern California, complete with golf stories to wow her. Even though she was never a golfer, she knows that my husband and I golf, and she listened intently. Then she asked about Oliver (her deceased brother) and about what he did while we were gone. I knew that she meant our son Evan, so I updated her on all of his comings and goings.

She then sighed again, rubbing her forehead over and over. She was so worried. What about? I sat down and prepared to wait and listen as she tried to describe the concern to me. It was the funeral, she said. She knew she missed her father's funeral, which was "over the dam," she informed me. But what about a visit to her mother? How could we work that out? She was concerned that she didn't know where her mother was living and thought maybe she might be living with Edith (my mother, her sister). Did I think that they might be living together? Did I know where Edith lived?

We have had this similar conversation at every visit for the last few months. I have since forgotten the actual conversation, and with whom, that triggered this frantic thought that she missed her father's funeral and about what she could do now to rectify it. My approach with these conversations had been to listen, nod, sit, and wait while she rubbed her forehead and told me that she knew things weren't the greatest between her and her mother, but she really wanted to get out to Random Lake, Wisconsin, to visit her.

As in all previous conversations, after about twenty minutes, I would very quietly tell her that she did such a good job at Grandpa's funeral, arranging the service and the meal and asking all the male members of the family to be the pallbearers — that it was a very wonderful family event and Grandma was so grateful. I also told her that she did the same thing when Grandma died. The family could not have arranged those funerals without her leadership. She began rubbing her forehead with two hands now, looked at me, and said, "Oh no. I don't remember any of that."

We sat in silence for about four minutes. It seemed forever. People, carts, and wheelchairs passed by the room every five seconds while we sat. Silent. Finally, I ended it, deftly changing the subject, saying, "Mamie, I am so glad that you enjoy the Penelope meetings!"

She picked her head up off her chest, dropped her hands from rubbing her forehead, looked straight at me with amazingly clear eyes, and said, "Oh that is a *fine* gathering. It is very well thought out. And it is turning into something so important." She continued slowly, as she was searching for her thoughts, trying to put them in order:

> You know that I have not played the piano at all since I moved here. [Mamie had a seventy-four-year career as a single woman running her own business as a piano teacher.] I was thinking that this event probably wouldn't be the time to start, but they surely will need musicians for the production. I was thinking that there are many fine musicians that live here, but it makes me think about practicing.

Mamie then told me a long, complicated, hard-to-follow story about a childhood friend, Lucille, who is also living here now, at Luther Manor. Lucille is also in the Penelope discussion group. Lucille told a story about their childhood in Random Lake and Lucille's family grocery store. Mamie said it was a nice story. "She respected me, and it contributed to the discussion, even though she sometimes treats me like a little sister." I laughed as I told Mamie that, in fact, Lucille is two years older, so Mamie could be a younger sister, but that since Mamie was so used to being the older sister in her family, I'm sure that could be difficult!

Thanks to Penelope, we were able to laugh, hug, kiss, and enjoy each other and end our visit with smiles all around. In my wildest dreams about this

Penelope Project, I never thought about the personal takeaway that I would get. I never thought about how personally these experiences would affect the residents, their families, and staff. And shame on me — the person-centered care advocate, forgetting that after all is said and done . . . it is all about the personal.

ON PLAYING THE SUITORS: IN DIALOGUE
Daniel Cohen and Rusty Tym

Daniel: Tell the story of how you came to be involved with the project. What made you want to do it?

Rusty: A poster on an easel in the Terrace lobby entrance of Luther Manor caught my eye and curiosity. It invited the residents to become part of a play. Upon realizing this project would be created through the synergy of Luther Manor, UWM, and a professional acting group, I wanted to find out more.

Inquisitiveness usually leads to discovery, and once I learned the objectives of this project, I wanted to be invested. Having only been involved in one play in my life [Horace Vandergelder in *Hello, Dolly!* in Waukesha Theatre, 1982] the itch was there. Now I wanted to scratch it again.

Daniel: What was the hardest for you?

Rusty: I walked into the first discussion group, and to my surprise [there] were two video cameramen and a lady with a boom microphone along with several residents of Luther Manor in attendance. The visual recording captured our every word and movement. I was simply expecting a script with a speaking part. Yet the discussion centered on our experiences. I did not realize how expansive this project was going to be until that first introductory process. The hardest thing for me about this project was these meetings. I wanted to plunge right into the play and find my part in it all. Meeting after meeting, our discussions meandered through people's experiences with patience, conviction, uncertainty, and adeptness. We were asked to imagine what the characters would look like, as a UWM student sketched our description. I was bored and impatient to get going, not realizing that we were slowly but surely becoming a vital part of fleshing out the characters, the plot, and the process for the anatomy of the play. It was a valuable lesson for me to encounter this profound method of creativity. In addition, I found new friends and discovered a hidden fondness for them. I never realized before how much socializing was a part of me. I have always been a curious person, and how wonderfully fascinating it was to learn about so many other people's life experiences and how uniquely they filtered into the storytelling process. The hardest part of the project became the easiest, and I began to eagerly look forward to subsequent gatherings.

Daniel: What did you get out of it? What did you gain from being involved?

Rusty: I gained so much from my involvement. This golden opportunity came to Luther Manor, and it would be well worth the time, energy, and perseverance for me to seize the moment and absorb it. I was surrounded by gifted people — dramatists, learned professors, exceptional Luther Manor staff — all offering their experiences, energies, and backgrounds to foster our potential in the arts. Their dynamism surrounded us. So I watched the process, ingested the atmosphere, studied the people, imitated their enthusiasm, and gained valuable confidence. I was feeling like I fit in, I belonged in this environment. My appetite for more just beginning.

Daniel: You continued to incorporate drama and storytelling at Luther Manor — can you talk a bit about that? What felt important about that?

Rusty: *Finding Penelope* created a foundation of confidence among some of the residents of Luther Manor. The staff recognized this and created a committee called Beyond Penelope. The discussions centered on how we can continue the arts and storytelling within our campus. How can we incorporate what we absorbed for future benefit? Timidly, I suggested that since memorizing was a huge drawback, we try to create a radio stage play. This way the cast could merely read their script in front of a microphone and audience. Except for doing it here at Luther Manor, it is nothing new. What would make our efforts unique is that the residents would write, stage, and fabricate the final product all within the confines of our campus.

So with the valuable and remarkable cooperation of resource managers Linda Moscicki and Kathi Brueggemann, I formed WLM Radio. Luther Manor was so very supportive of the idea that they donated a two-bedroom apartment for rehearsals. Our pretend frequency became F101 [instead of FM 101] because the apartment number was, you guessed it, F101.

Based on the astonishing results of *Finding Penelope*'s discussion groups, we held several focus groups with Terrace residents. Always a packed meeting, we developed the script from ideas that poured forth from many inventive minds. I encouraged people to submit their own skit ideas, and soon we had a show. Actually we had enough material for a couple of shows. I had people stopping me in the hallways and submitting written skits or ideas for skits.

I directed our pilot show called *The Witty, the Wise, and the Weathered*. We staged several skits centered on the sillier side of life at [Luther Manor]. We learned a great deal and used that knowledge to make another play called *Schmaltz and Other Fond Memories*.

The enthusiasm from the Terrace residents manifested itself in their open display of true eagerness to do more. In another play, staged in May 2014, three different writers each created a murder mystery and competed with each other to have the audience select their version of the dastardly deed.

In addition, F101 studios will be transformed to look like a radio station complete with seating for an audience. There we plan on presenting recreations of old radio shows like Jack Benny, Abbot and Costello, *Inner Sanctum*, etc. With a generous donation from a couple of TV stations we now have a complete TV production studio. We plan on videotaping all our mini-presentations for future broadcasting on Luther Manor's closed-circuit system.

It is fully evident that those involved have opened themselves up to an experience of enrichment. I have witnessed their individual acting prowess, their improved skills, and their unbounded enthusiasm toward their writing endeavors. Penelope lives on right here where her original concept kicked up a rumpus. There is a need for individuals to further express themselves [no matter what age], to have a feeling of belonging and contributing, and most importantly, knowing you make a difference. It's happening here at Luther Manor, thanks to all who helped find Penelope.

OK, now you. How did you get involved with the project? Why did you want to do it?

Daniel: I worked with the Sojourn Theatre on a previous production in Oregon called *On the Table*. That process was such a unique blend of challenge and reward that I seized the opportunity to work with the Sojourn team again. I was also very interested in working within a senior living community. My grandmother spent the last years of her life in a nursing home, and I spent many hours there with her. After she passed away, I returned to the facility to write a paper about it for a high school English class. I hadn't been in the building for at least a year, but I was immediately stopped by a nurse who approached me with a pleasantly pensive look on her face. "Marian Cohen, room 203," she said. I was speechless, but my expression prompted her to explain that she recognized me from my childhood photos on Grandma's nightstand. I could not believe that a caregiver had come to know my grandmother so fully and to carry her in memory after over a year. That's when I learned that such facilities, given the many profound purposes they serve, are inherently fascinating places. Between the chance to work with Sojourn and my own personal history with elder care communities, Penelope was a project I didn't want to miss.

Rusty: What was the hardest thing for you?

Daniel: The hardest part of the project for me was probably developing ["devising"] the script. We were working with so many important metaphors that, at times, I struggled to be clear in my head about what story we were telling. Specifically, I remember seemingly endless discussions about the final scene and the reveal of Penelope. Would one actor play Penelope? Would every actor play Penelope? Would no actor play Penelope? Would we cast the audience as Penelope? Would a sock puppet play Penelope [it may well have come up in a particularly delirious moment]? Each choice would tell a very different story; Penelope could be a real person, could exist inside all of us, could be an idea, could be an illusion. By choosing Joyce Heinrich [Luther Manor resident] to play Penelope before a chorus, underscoring her text with movement, we seemed to combine several ideas of what "Penelope" was and is. At first, I was stubbornly dedicated to coming up with a nice, clean metaphor. By the end of the process, I came to understand that the whole theatrical event the audience experienced could never be bound by one simple narrative or idea. The "problems" we had during this part of the process were fantastic ones to have and are only made possible by tireless, curious, and humble guides like Anne and Maureen, who are game to try anything that might enrich the story.

Rusty: What did you get out of it? What did you gain?

Daniel: I gained an appreciation for how willing folks are to play, to be silly, to attempt exhausting and uncomfortable new things. I still draw inspiration from watching the Luther Manor staff continually say yes to each step of the project. Throughout the play-development process, I gained a new capacity to sit with unanswered questions and a newly found trust that the play would reveal itself to us over time. I gained friends.

Perhaps most importantly, Penelope shifted my thinking about elders. My time at Luther Manor made me realize that I have few genuine relationships with older people. Prior to Penelope, my interactions with elders relied on an awkward, forced reverence, while my interactions *about* older people, amongst peers, relied on cheap jokes ridiculing hearing loss, dementia, etc. Penelope showed me that both attitudes are merely different forms of distancing people of different generations. I grew interested in fostering intergenerational friendships not as the important work of receiving the torch from the bearers of history but simply as loving, joyful, human connections. Daily life makes this hard; I don't interact with many folks much older than my parents. But in the few intergenerational relationships I have started to build since Penelope, I feel the impact of the project very greatly indeed.

ON PLAYING PENELOPE: IN DIALOGUE
Joyce Heinrich and Nikki Zaleski

Joyce: I look back at those first days of the Penelope Project and remember how I wondered what ever possessed me to try being in theatre for the first time at the age of eighty-one. What was I thinking? I knew that all of you from the Sojourn group were well versed in things of the theatre — things like endless rehearsals and memorizing parts.

Nikki: I felt an identical anxiety! At the time we began Penelope, I saw myself as a writer, director, and theatre-maker in general but hadn't worked my performance muscles in some time. In all honesty, Joyce, I was sure you would upstage me by miles. I brought an intense fear of failure to the Penelope Project with me. I was afraid of not doing justice to the epic stories of Luther Manor. I was afraid of negatively disrupting the lives of residents. I was afraid of stirring an otherwise settled pot and not being present to clean up the mess later. Your humor and constant reminding of the power of our work helped me overcome that fear.

Joyce: I had seen the script, and to be very honest, I just didn't "get it." Then I realized I was just taking the role of a maid. I had one scene and about eight words. I guessed I would be up to doing that. I could not grasp what the Penelope Project would come to mean to me. I remember that first meeting.

Nikki: Yes! That first meeting. Anne Basting described her near-ten-year relationship with Luther Manor. Maureen Towey set the tone for the project. The Luther Manor staff blew me away with their thoughtful and spot-on questions about the piece. And then you and Rusty Tym introduced yourselves. Your wit, history, and courage took all of about ninety seconds to become clear, and I thought, "Well, this is going to be good."

Joyce: Oh, you were all so young. You treated us with such respect. We were all so very quiet, polite, and a bit distant. That would all change in the coming weeks as we bonded. Do you remember the constant changes made to the script?

Nikki: Of course! Though painful at times, the script changes actually made up my favorite part of the playmaking process. I learned so much from the way Anne tuned into rehearsals and discoveries at Luther Manor. She had a clear vision for the overall structure but remained open to stories as they emerged from rehearsal walls.

Joyce: Yes, Anne always reminded us this was a work in progress. I felt as if I came alive when I was with all of you. All this was in the beginning. My role had expanded from that of a maid into being Penelope. I was a bit overwhelmed by the rapid changes in the script, but all of the younger people kept me coming back for more.

Nikki: Joyce, I felt so similarly about you, Rusty, and the other older adults I grew close to at Luther Manor. In the moments when the material felt too heavy, or the Milwaukee winter too cold, or rehearsals too long, or death too present, the relationships I formed with residents offered the strongest tonic for burnout. These relationships were not a sidebar to the project itself — they were core to the success of Penelope. In other plays I've worked on, casts grew close as a result of spending extended time together. In Penelope, we grew together because the material made us. Forming authentic relationships, especially with the actors living with Alzheimer's and dementia, was a necessity of being present and fluid together on stage.

Joyce: Nikki, a quitter I am not, but one day I had made up my mind that I was leaving the Penelope Project — enough of these rehearsals in a play I did not understand. I had been at every meeting. I had heard more than enough about Odysseus. I loved the young actors from UWM and Sojourn Theatre, but I must tell them this very day that I was dropping out. I carefully rehearsed the words I would use as we gathered at what was to be my last rehearsal with them. And then it happened. We were entering the Health Care Center to do one of the scenes. As always, there was a cluster of residents gathered in a semicircle waiting for something, anything, to happen. It was then that a young actor, Daniel Cohen, entered. He walked slowly across the room to one of the wheelchairs. He quietly knelt down in front of the chair, looked into the lady's eyes, took her hand, and began to speak. Then the transformation began as her eyes twinkled and her lips moved. As a witness to that moment, I realized that this is what the Penelope Project was all about. It was in that moment that I, too, was transformed. Never again did I think of quitting. I became a committed and a new Penelope.

Nikki: I loved hearing this story, Joyce, and remember others like it. Soon after the close of Penelope, much was discussed about how meaningful the project was for Luther Manor residents. I don't think we spoke enough about how the piece transformed the UWM and Sojourn participants.

My grandmother passed away from Alzheimer's seven months before the Penelope Project. I was afraid of her illness, afraid to talk to her in the last few months of her life, afraid of her aging, afraid of her death. Penelope helped me understand this fear and the misassumption that my grandmother wouldn't understand me in the last few months of her life. Like I feared upsetting Luther Manor residents, I feared distressing, confusing, or panicking my grandmother. I remember pleading with Anne one rehearsal: "Please give us some training on how to talk to people with Alzheimer's." "Practice and be present," she responded. And you! I remember asking you one rehearsal if you thought we were negatively impacting the lives of any of the residents. Were we annoying them? Frustrating them? Distressing them? You insisted we were better than TV. You insisted that we inspired and interested them. You insisted that we brought them joy. You kept me in the project again and again with this insistence. Penelope positioned younger adults in partnership with our elders. It helped move us past any fear or stigma related to aging and rooted us in powerful connections to each other. This change will forever affect my relationships with my family, with other elders, and to my own aging process.

Joyce: I can't believe how much I grew during the final weeks of rehearsal. I caught the magic that was going on all around me. I finally understood what the Penelope Project was accomplishing—how it bonded the younger and older generations. We had such a relationship, Nikki. On a more personal level, I have changed a lot from that first day when I was so very frightened by what I had gotten myself into. Since my experience in Penelope, I acted in three more plays. One of the plays again bridged the generation gap by including young schoolchildren, many of whom came from the inner city of Milwaukee and were also discovering the importance of the creative arts. We have started a theatre group here at Luther Manor, and I have also been able to take a creative writing course right here. I even wrote a murder mystery. All this from the seeds of knowing people like you, Nikki, and all the other Penelope participants.

FIVE SECONDS AFTER THE AUDIENCE LEFT
Anne Basting

Unfortunately, no one who saw the performance could see one of my very favorite parts of it. Each of the five scenes in *Finding Penelope* took place in high-traffic locations at Luther Manor — the Health Care Center dining area, the Faith and Education Center, the Welcome Center, and the dining room of the Courtyards. In each location, there was a crew waiting to strike the scene as soon as the last audience member was no longer visible. In each space, a team of students, faculty, and Luther Manor staff and residents waited to spring into action. In the Health Care Center we were like a well-seasoned pit crew disassembling the large weaving that hung above what was the Weavers' Scene, and we would shortly return to the dining area. When audiences arrived next in the Welcome Center, they would see up to forty chairs gathered around the hearth. As soon as the back of the last audience member disappeared around the corner, following the old beggar (also known as Odysseus) singing "Rambling Man" through the hallways, another team daisy-chained every last chair back to its original position around the conference table down the hall or into the four-top formation in the adjacent sitting area.

The Courtyards dining hall, also known as the location for the Banquet Scene in which 108 suitors would be slaughtered, was the most difficult of all the rapid strikes. We finished the scene just thirty minutes before supper time. The set demanded that we rearrange most of the tables and throw 108 coats (representing the 108 suitors) over the chairs (and in the air and on the ground). Scores of black and silver balloons created both a festive and an ominous atmosphere. Tables would need to be rearranged into exactly the right spot and set with specific dining instructions/needs for specific residents. This area is akin to "assisted living," where a high percentage of the residents are wrestling with some form of memory loss. Routine is essential. Meal staff is paid by the hour. Luther Manor agreed to let us perform the scene there only when we assured them that our team would ensure the strike happened properly and supper would not be delayed.

I was unable to stay and help with this scene strike as I was needed in the next and final scene. We always preset the final scene, which took place on the transept area in the Faith and Education Center, with enough chairs for the ticketed audience members on each day. The idea was to make each audience member feel there was a place just for him or her — no empty seats. But the show developed a "pied piper" effect, and we always needed more chairs for the people who followed the performance as it went through the halls of Luther Manor and joined us for the climax. Sometimes this meant arranging an additional twenty to thirty chairs in a careful arc facing the stage.

Though I couldn't stay to see the magic of the strike in the dining hall, one of my favorite memories of the performance came from participating in the strike in scene 3, the Welcome Center. There were four of us who informally became the Welcome Center strike team. Julianne was Luther Manor's receptionist who sat at the desk throughout the scene doing her job. We incorporated her opening line ("Luther Manor, how may I direct your call?") into the scene. Ryan was a student in the theatre production class. On the second day of the performances, the daisy chain was particularly effective. Chairs slid so easily from one person to the next, down the hall into the conference room, that I started to laugh — the joy of efficiency bubbled over. Only then did I make a conscious note of the fourth team member who was sliding chairs in my direction. It was Dave Beinlich, the administrator of the Health Care Center and Courtyards. It was the boss. He was laughing too. Clearly, Dave, Julianne, Ryan, and I were quite a team, putting on a great show. Too bad the audience was already gone.

THE MAGIC OF THE MOVEMENT
Anne Basting and Leonard Cruz

The *Odyssey* is a story of war, wandering, waiting, and welcoming. Penelope stands apart from other Greek heroines because she does manage successfully to wait for Odysseus and she warmly welcomes strangers into her home (following the Greek codes of hospitality). As part of the devising process, the arts team aimed to create a "Welcome Dance" to be used by the chorus in the final scene to welcome Odysseus back home.

Welcoming the stranger is a very loaded metaphor in long-term care settings. In some situations, the stranger might be an outside visitor. It might be a new resident. In some ways, the person in the mirror might seem a stranger to you. A person might identify with his or her thirty- or forty- or fifty-year-old self—and see the older person he or she has become, possibly with some serious disabilities, as a stranger. Can one welcome one's self as a stranger? Welcoming the stranger in this sense is to welcome and accept one's changing self.

After their weeklong January residency, the Sojourn team flew off to their various homes and would return in three weeks for the final push—two weeks of devising and rehearsal, and two weeks of performances. In the meantime, we (local residents, staff, students, and artists) had a list of "challenges" to accomplish. One such challenge was to create the "Welcome Dance" for the scene in which Penelope finally recognizes and welcomes Odysseus home after his twenty-year absence.

We had the uncanny good fortune of being joined by Leonard Cruz, who was nearing the end of his PhD studies in urban education at UWM. Leonard saw our flier hanging in the Peck School of the Arts building and was drawn by our project's focus on community outreach, in which he himself has experience, specifically in urban education. Leonard came to the Sojourn Workshop for UWM students in October of 2010, and we encouraged him to attend the audition that afternoon. In the course of his audition, we learned that Leonard had danced with Pina Bausch (world-renowned German dancer, choreographer, and teacher) as well as Bill T. Jones (American artistic director, choreographer, and dancer) and had worked with nondancers with disabilities in urban and special needs communities. His class schedule prohibited him from participating in the play itself, but he was able to join me at Luther Manor during February 2011 to work with staff and residents to find and hone the "Welcome Dance."

For Leonard's first visit to Luther Manor I asked him simply to introduce himself to the four different care areas. He remembers his first impression of Luther Manor as being warm, welcoming, and positive. We started in the Adult Day Center. Wearing his "Hawaiian Punch" T-shirt, Leonard introduced himself by teaching a few gestures from Hawaiian folk dance, which he performed as a child with his family and later taught in urban workshops to children who weren't familiar with Pacific Island cultures. When teaching gestures, says Leonard, "it is important to transform oneself into the very essence of the dance movements."

Cruz began with gestures of natural elements: "Water," "Mountain," "Palm Tree," "Rainbow," "Wind," "Rain." About a dozen Day Center participants gathered in a semicircle and repeated his movements. They eagerly learned the gestures for feeling senses: "Heart/Love," "Spirit," "Home." They repeated them with so much grace and asked for more. Leonard taught them "Fish," "Bird," and sensory actions: "Calling You," "Hearing You," "Seeing You." The number of participants started to grow. Staff gathered around as well with great interest. Suddenly, there were forty-five participants and a dozen staff and volunteers, doing every Hawaiian gesture that Leonard knew, returning his movements with just as much emotion. He looked at me in a bit of a panic: "They want more," he said, "and that's all there is!"

There was a giddiness in the room. We would call out the name of a gesture, and the large group would do it. We would call out a sequence. They would do it. Nearly everyone in the Day Center was now gathered around us. Leonard remarked that the moment was flowering with the *ohana* spirit of family and love.

The residents were still hungry for more. I suggested that they tell stories with the gestures. One man told a story of growing up in a house by a river and fishing and canoeing and listening to birds. I remembered our eventual purpose — to find the "Welcome Dance" — and asked them, "How would you show a stranger that they are welcome in your home?" Richard, a participant seated in the front row, offered following sequence:

My heart
Is open to you
My soul/spirit
Welcomes you

To my home
I am calling you
I am hearing you
I am seeing you
Your eyes sparkle
Like the stars

The group cheered. We repeated it together. Richard had given a beautiful gift to the group, and we returned it to him by echoing his sentiment. Leonard was amazed by how responsive and expressive all of the residents were to the gestures he taught them, and even more so by their improvisational spirit, which rang true for Leonard. "In Hawaiian folk dance, most dances are improvised or uniquely planned out with what the dancer wants to share and communicate with their audience," he said.

Our simple introduction of Leonard to the residents and participants of Luther Manor yielded more than we could have hoped for. We thanked everyone and moved to the hallway to make our way to the Health Care Center. But we had to pause — what just happened? Was that normal? No, I told him. That was magical. There is something about the gestural language and something about you — your warmth, your love, your openness — that they are responding to.

Leonard said that the experience went both ways — that because the residents were so open with wanting to express their feelings and warmth with him, he was in turn lifted up. "It's their desire to express, to communicate — it's something that they're missing in their lives," he said.

Over the course of the next three weeks Leonard and I visited all four areas of care. To our surprise, we ran into residents with personal stories of Hawaiian trips and previous encounters with the folk dance forms. We visited people one-on-one over lunch in the dining rooms. Each time, we taught people a few basic gestures and then Richard's elegant "Welcome Dance." In the Health Care Center, there were people with serious physical and cognitive disabilities who opened to the warmth of that "Welcome Dance" and responded, sometimes with tremendous effort, with whatever abilities they had. Some couldn't raise their arms above their heads for the gesture of "Home." "It doesn't matter," said Leonard. "It has the same meaning. It's beautiful anyway." And it was. The staff could sense it too — an almost pure sense of giving, of love. They did not quite feel comfortable enough to join us, but they watched, mouths and eyes wide, sensing the gifts coming from the residents.

My heart
Is open to you
My soul/spirit
Welcomes you
To my Home
I am calling you
I am hearing you
I am seeing you
Your eyes
Sparkle
Like the stars

On the ride home in the car with Leonard on that first day, we felt euphoric from the exchanges we'd had. We traded stories of "Did you see . . . ? Did you feel . . . ?" Yes. Yes. Me too. I remarked on how much he was sweating during the simple movements—was it hard work? "No!" he said. "They were giving me so much love! It was overwhelming. And it was cathartic, because of the hunger of wanting to reach out from both sides." Leonard, who was aching to return to performance and dance after his strenuous PhD program, felt a connection to the residents. It was a moment of spiritual and physical healing.

Over the next couple of weeks, I photographed Leonard doing the various gestures so we would remember them. I didn't need to worry. There is clearly something about the gestures that stays in the body, mind, and spirit. People would walk up to Leonard and do the gestures in greeting. Even weeks later, the residents and participants could do all forty-five that he taught them. We know that we will never forget them.

FINDING AN ENDING
Maureen Towey

One hundred people, we kept saying. A chorus of one hundred Luther Manor residents would be the end of our play. The idea of Penelope would be spread across the human landscape of Luther Manor, collectively reimagining the act of waiting and weaving. The Luther Manor staff gently pointed out some clear obstacles for our choral dreams. The health of many of the residents changes from day to day, so they can't commit to rehearsing or performing every day. In addition, many residents have memory issues, so memorizing text would be difficult, if not impossible. Even for the independent residents who did not have major memory issues, they were put off by the idea of memorizing at all.

We had a breakthrough with our ideas for the chorus when Leonard, our choreographer, came to Luther Manor with the goal of creating a "Welcome Dance" for the final scene. As he modeled the gestural language to residents, they quickly took it up as their own, helping us to realize that the chorus could be almost completely nonverbal. (See the chapter "The Magic of the Movement" for more on this process.) No memorization was needed. Chorus members could simply be present and respond to a leader. Even those with limited range of movement could take the intention of the movement and run with it. In fact, their limitations simply became variations that made the movements more personal and beautiful.

We took the ideas from Leonard's choreography sessions and incorporated them into the script. But this discovery alone would not make a great ending. We still had to stage it, frame their actions effectively, and wrap up the entire experience. The location for the finale, the Faith and Education Center, was a wide-open, fairly traditional space used for worship services and educational, social, and cultural events. We were resistant to using their "stage," a small area with strong icons and associations with the Lutheran services. We felt we were effectively blending fact and fiction, that we had thrust our audiences directly into a real, immersive place. So, we were nervous that putting our chorus on a stage would put them on display in a way that was not useful or that would hold strong affiliations with a church service. What other audience formations might maintain integrated, co-occupied space? Or could keep us physically with the story and the place?

Our initial idea was that the audience would be seated in the round and that the chorus of Penelopes would blend in with them. But as we attempted this staging, we got more and more lost. After two years of work and discoveries, we were two weeks from showtime, and we were still trying to find our ending.

Creating an ending is hairy in new work. To make a satisfying journey, you can't ignore the tug of resolution, both for the artist and for the audience. You want to stretch the muscle of the myth to its full extension. To negotiate but not manipulate emotion, you must harness as much truth as you can. We had all the right ingredients—in the high, hopeful stained-glass windows in the room, in this group of people from Luther Manor willing to put themselves in front of an audience's gaze, in the repetition of gestures and simple phrases that had been living rehearsal to the residents and staff who hosted us all these months. We just needed to wrangle it into an order and let it go. In this way, it could function not as some grand cathartic finale but as a humble, purposeful, and beautiful point on a continuum for everyone present.

After a particularly difficult day of rehearsal, Anne Basting, Shannon Scrofano, and I went, literally, back to the drawing board. Sitting in Anne's living room with two huge whiteboards in front of us, we were able to sketch out both the dialogue and the staging for the end. We wish there was more of a science to this—for the three of us, we simply go through enough wrong ideas that we eventually find our way to the right one. This requires being comfortable with uncertainty for an extended period. As director, I was often the one who kept conceptual thinking in line with logistics—if we dreamt for too long, we may not have left ourselves enough time to execute well. Shannon functioned as more than a designer—in addition to tending to the space, she was our best conceptual problem solver. Anne wrote the words but also maintained an acute sensitivity to how the audience was being engaged. She insisted on the chorus, in part, because it meant the best way to experience the performance was to be a part of it.

The two story lines—Odysseus' journey to find and be recognized by Penelope, and Mira's journey to find and be accepted by her mother—were lining up. The audience's journey paralleled them both—literally going from "stranger" (written on their nametags) to welcomed members of the chorus/community. They would be recognized and welcomed by Penelope as well.

Despite our initial hesitation, it was clear that being on the stage was meaningful for the residents, their families, and the staff. With permission, we cleared off some of the church iconography so the stage became a more neutral space. Then CEO David Keller gave us permission to "call" the show on the public announcement system that went to the entire one-million-square-feet community. One of those "calls" was, *Penelope, you are at places in the F&E. Penelope, you are at places.* This meant that anyone in the entire community who wanted to play Penelope should come down to the F&E (Faith and Education Center) at that time. It was a moment of enormous trust. Who would come that day? Would anyone? Audience members (as they walked from one scene to another) didn't realize that the people they were passing in the hallways were actually on their way to the F&E to play in the final chorus. The "Penelopes" they were "looking for" were passing them in the halls. They were right in front of them.

The ending of the performance is the scene that we feel most proud of, both conceptually and in terms of community engagement. We did end up using the stage, and it was exactly the right choice. We never quite had one hundred people in the chorus, but the stage always felt perfectly full. The text of the final scene ended up being primarily words we had already found—words from the residents, words from the *Odyssey*—just ordered in a new way and bringing project and play to an emotional close. Sometimes, the brightest moments of performance are the most difficult to find, and the most effective forms of community engagement demand trial and error that ends only when—it ends.

EXCERPT FROM *Finding Penelope*, SCENE 5
Anne Basting

SCENE 5

*OLD NURSE laughs and helps him with the curtain. There is a group of 30+
people (staff, residents, family, friends of Luther Manor) gathered in rows of
semicircles on stage, facing the STRANGERS.*

*STAFF (DANIEL, RUSTY, MAGGIE, GLEN, JULIA) are with them,
making slow-motion welcoming gestures. SOUL AND SPIRIT. I SEE YOU.
NIKKI is seated in front of them, guiding their movements and lines.*

*MIRA talks to her Mother. ODYSSEUS talks to the group playing
PENELOPE.*

*JOYCE speaks to MIRA. PENELOPES speak to ODYSSEUS. NURSE can
speak to everyone.*

JOYCE/PENELOPE P.
Hello Dear.

STAFF gestures: I am calling you. Soul and spirit.

MIRA
Hi Mom.

ODYSSEUS
My dear Penelope.

MIRA
Mom. I'm sorry.

MIRA AND ODYSSEUS
I didn't mean to be away so long.

ODYSSEUS
There were just — so — many — monsters.

MIRA
I had to prove to myself that I could do it. I had to — Mom?

JOYCE/PENELOPE P.
Hello Dear.

MIRA
It's Mira.

STAFF gestures: I am calling you. Soul and spirit (continued rolling, symbolizing PENELOPE/PENELOPES).

JOYCE/PENELOPE P.
That's a pretty name.

ODYSSEUS
At long last we have returned to you. (*No response.*) Penelope? (*No response.*)
PENELOPE?

STAFF gestures: I AM CALLING YOU. I AM CALLING YOU! My soul and spirit.

MIRA AND ODYSSEUS
Do you know me?

JOYCE/PENELOPE P.
Do you know me?

ODYSSEUS
Do I — know you? Do I know you?? Oh Nurse. Nurse. To come so far. And now. I fear I am mortally wounded.

OLD NURSE
You've been gone a long time my boy. Prove yourself to her.

JOYCE struggles with her knitting.

MIRA
Can I help you?

JOYCE hands her a skein of yarn.

JOYCE/PENELOPE P.
Thank you. Have we met?

MIRA
You are my cunning, noble, wise, and lovely Penelope.

JOYCE
(*gently laughing*) Oh . . . I wouldn't say that about myself.

ODYSSEUS
(*The following moves from ODYSSEUS saying it in despair to his realization that he knows them all — from observing them during the play — and that this is how he will prove himself to "her."*)
Do I know you?
You are my cunning, noble, wise, and lovely Queen.

You make Ithaca home for me.

STAFF is guiding PENELOPE through the Welcome Dance gestures, very slowly.

You are the one that made a cake shaped like a castle.

You are the one that played "Sentimental Journey."

You are the one that did this. . . . (*hand gesture of crying*)

You are the one that dances with your walker.

You are the one that simply beams when I see you in the hallway.

You are the one that knits multicolored socks.

You are the one that went from four little suitcases to a four-bedroom house.

You are the one that helped us make the Welcome Dance.

You are the one that that speaks Hungarian.

You are the one that loves the little birds.

You are the one that plays Sheepshead to win.

You are the one that said that being part of this project helped you feel like you belong to something.

You are the one that answers the phone, "Luther Manor, how may I direct your call?"

You are the one that said, "At home there will always be chocolate."

You are the one that wore the beautiful sari to the years of service dinner.

You are the one that passed away last Tuesday.

You are the one that held her hand.

You are the one that wanted to play the Cyclops.

You are the one that has an organ in your room, but can no longer play.

You are the one that fought in the Korean War.

You are the one that visits her husband in the nursing home every day.

You are the one that traveled the world.

You are the ones that have been married for sixty-two years.

You are the one that is a professional drummer.

You are the one with a PhD in French History.

You are the one who tells stories of parakeets.

You are the one that taught piano your whole life.

You, you are the ones that make this place home.

OLD NURSE

And so says the *Odyssey*, Penelope felt her knees go slack, her heart surrender, recognizing the strong, clear signs he offered. She dissolved in tears and welcomed him home.

OLD NURSE speaks. She and STAFF guide the PENELOPES in the Welcome Dance.

OLD NURSE
My heart is open to you. My soul and my spirit welcome you home. I am calling you. (*PENELOPES do movement.*)

ODYSSEUS
I am hearing you. (*with movement*)

OLD NURSE
I am seeing you. (*PENELOPES do movement.*)

ODYSSEUS
I am seeing you. (*with movement*) Your eyes, my beloved, sparkle like stars.

Penelope has come to signify all the heroes/heroines along life's pathway:

- those who have the patience to listen with their hearts
- those who wait for me to figure things out
- those who rejoice with me when I do
- those who love me in spite of my warts—or maybe sometimes because of them!
- those who identify the silver linings in life's challenges and re-frame circumstance to find the lessons to be learned
- those who know how to laugh and have a good time
- those who allow life to unfold rather than force life to fit into their "plan" for it
- those who figure out what to do with themselves while life is unfolding
- those who embrace the talents and gifts of all people.

—Linda Moscicki, Social Worker, Luther Manor Terrace

What happened as a result of the process of creating the Penelope Project? Was there any lasting impact for the residents? The staff? The students? The artists? As a team, it was important to us to match the rigor of the art-making process and the care process with a rigorous evaluation. We applied for Institutional Review Board approval for our study and wrapped surveys, interviews, and focus group discussions around the entire process.

Some of the results of reflections, interviews, and focus groups are peppered throughout the book. This section shares the results of the evaluation more deeply, with an eye on the 360-degree impact of the project—on families, staff, students, volunteers, residents, and artists alike. This section also contains essays that address what happened after the play closed and the unique challenges of ending projects like Penelope. When such powerful relationships are built during the act of creation, how do you stop?

BEYOND PENELOPE AT LUTHER MANOR
Ellie Rose

Luther Manor was bursting with new energy while preparing and putting on *Finding Penelope*. There were strangers in our halls, weaving on the walls, and laughter in the dining rooms. We didn't want the excitement to end. Soon, however, we started to wonder, what was going to happen after UWM and Sojourn partners left?

A focus group of life enrichment specialists met once per month during the Penelope Project to share stories, problem solve, and communicate action plans. Each care area (the Terrace, Courtyards, Health Care Center, Adult Day Center, and even Volunteer Services) had a representative at each meeting. At our last meeting, we had an intimate discussion about the Penelope we had become. It was us — we who had learned how to make Penelope more than a mythical story. It was us — we who had learned how to collaborate with a larger community. *Finding Penelope* may have ended, but the Penelope Project did not have to stop there. As a result, we all agreed we did not want to go back to the old way of segregated life-enrichment programs. We wanted to use the valuable skills we all brought to the table and create programs that invited creative engagement from everyone in our community.

Since *Finding Penelope*, the Luther Manor community has implemented multiple cross-department programs. We reinstalled the weaving in the Faith and Education Center lobby and the Adult Day Center gallery. We collaborated with the Modjeska Theatre Company, a local group that works with underserved schoolchildren, to stage *Now I Can Soar*, an intergenerational theatrical production. We held creative writing workshops, which yielded writing used in two original, resident-directed plays: the *The Witty, the Wise, and the Weathered* and *Schmaltz and Other Fond Memories* theatrical productions. We collaborated with renowned children's theatre First Stage on an original, intergenerational production in 2015. In the realm of visual art, we partnered with the local chapter of the Alzheimer's Association in the Memories in the Making program to create expressive watercolor paintings with residents and participants. Working with UWM faculty, we helped design the curriculum for, teach, and participate in "CREATE/CHANGE: Transforming Care for Elders through Creative Engagement," a summer institute at UWM for artists and care providers offered in 2012 and again in

2014. Guided by Rusty Tym (who played the suitors in *Finding Penelope*), residents and staff collaborated to form F101 WLM Radio, Luther Manor's authentic radio theatre productions group, which then created and staged the two original works mentioned above, *The Witty, the Wise, and the Weathered* and *Schmaltz and Other Fond Memories*.

Together, Rusty Tym, Joyce Heinrich, and I reflected on Beyond Penelope's progress and challenges.

Rusty: It's been challenging to lead focus groups, plan the next meeting, talk with staff, and inspire participation from everyone. I definitely feel like I have a purpose . . . thanks a lot, Penelope! The first WLM radio focus group was packed full! There were more questions than I had answers for. I was so excited and inspired to continue leading. But then it got difficult. The groups were smaller, and less people were able to visualize how they could contribute. I wanted to invite the other departments, but I didn't know what they would do and I could not take on another meeting.

Joyce: I've tried to lead the book-reading groups, but only fifteen people come.

Ellie: Only? Fifteen people seems like a lot to me. How many people do you want to come?

Joyce: I would like to think that even though the reading group is not a theatrical performance at least thirty people would come.

Rusty: But I have noticed that the small groups are so much easier to lead. The discussions are deeper, more creative even. We get through more material and have a plan before we leave. I think there is value to these small groups.

Ellie: I agree, Rusty. So, if there are more smaller groups, how could each smaller group contribute to a larger project?

Rusty: Well . . . we are Penelope! Aren't we? We already know how.

ON THE CHALLENGES OF CONTINUITY IN
CIVIC ARTS PROJECTS: IN DIALOGUE
Michael Rohd and Anne Basting

Anne: There is clearly a desire among artists, their partners, and funding partners that projects like Penelope have some kind of lasting impact. As you
and I talked about Penelope's lasting impact, we began to wonder about
that desire itself. Is lasting impact necessary? Is it always a desire? [This exchange, which happened by email, is part of that exploration.]

Michael: One of the things that made the work on Penelope possible was the
history you had with Luther Manor. Through your previous work with
TimeSlips Creative Storytelling, and your relationship with Beth Meyer-
Arnold, there was both some mutual trust and a sense of how the place
functioned. There was much to learn, as we found out, but because of you,
there was more than a foot in the door. And this now carries forward. You
continue a relationship with Luther Manor, and Penelope continues to
have presence and impact there. So a question I have for you — and this
relates to a lot of Sojourn's work, which is highly present for a long period
of time, but not always indefinite — the question is, do you believe that for
arts-based practice to have impact in community, non-arts settings, there
has to be a certain commitment to a durational relationship leading up to
and beyond arts activity? In your mind, is true civic meaning only possible
when there isn't a firm endpoint to the work and the partnership?

Anne: True civic meaning — that is the holy grail indeed. I think true civic
meaning is possible with a combination of transparency and clear, mutual,
and achievable goal setting that extends the "project" period to include the
development, execution, and continuity phases. In studying other civic
arts projects, I think artists and community partners sometimes have a
vague sense of the desire for a project to have lasting impact — but like
end-of-life care, it's uncomfortable to talk about the end and what happens after. I think partners can talk about the end without prescribing
what it will be. For Penelope, we knew there would be a play, but that was
it. Our partnership agreements mention "products" that would be shared,
but without articulating what they would be. And we created ways to capture the impact of the project that we could in turn share publicly (focus

groups, interviews, surveys). The magic ingredient seems to be a combination of clarity of goals for each phase and openness about what the outcomes will actually be. Does that hold true in your experiences?

Michael: It does, especially the magic ingredients being clarity of goals and openness. I think I'd add communication. It's certainly implied by what you are saying, but I'm thinking about something Laura Zabel at Springboard for the Arts in Saint Paul, Minnesota, says. To paraphrase, she says that too often we think a good partnership in arts-based work means super-profound long-term commitment upfront — sort of a "Hey, let's get married before we've even had a first date." She goes on to say that lots of great work can happen in the courtship phase. And it may not lead to marriage. It may be we date, a little or a lot; we do some good work; and we move on. And that can be just fine.

This really speaks to my interest in civic practice work, which I see as work in which artists deploy their assets in service to the needs of a non-arts partner as gleaned through listening, not presuming. My belief is that small-scale projects have value, build capacity, allow us to test aesthetic and engagement tactics, and build the scaffolding we need for the larger-scale, longer-term projects we often aspire toward. Penelope was, is, a big project. But if we really break it down, I'd say there are tactics, there are phases, that can be separated out from the whole and lifted into other contexts with the promise of civic meaning being a fair and legitimate promise — as much as one can promise anything in an arts-based process beyond one's intentions and transparency. Which brings me to this question for you — what do you feel you promised, if anything, and to whom, when you began this project, and did you deliver what you promised?

Anne: The "courtship period" as you describe it was focused on coming to an agreement about common goals and individual (to the various partner organizations) objectives. This was the first time I had done this as an articulated part of the process. Usually it happens in the hasty period between reading the call for proposals and submitting the grant. But this time, it happened as an articulated phase, and it allowed for much better courtship. The initial call to the table (as in "Hey, let's have lunch!") was to create a professional work of art together with Sojourn, UWM, and Luther Manor. By the end of the courtship period, we found a common goal we could all three work toward — improving the quality of life of those who live, work, and visit Luther Manor through art-making.

I haven't read about this type of articulated phase of goal and objective setting—likely because of the challenge of raising the funds to be able to cover that phase of the development process. Do you see this phase as becoming more valued by funders and art-makers in this field?

Michael: I think there is a growing understanding now that field-building and, therefore, capacity-building need to be priorities—that for funders and service organizations to prioritize civic work (be it described in their particular vocabulary as civic engagement, audience engagement, civic practice, or participation) they have to take on hosting conversations about skills, about impact, and about ethics. They have to put energy and resources into identifying best practices and bringing exemplary practitioners and projects to more visible platforms, and they have to make learning opportunities. The question becomes how different fields consider this responsibility across disciplines and sectors. You have been very involved, for years, in the health and the aging communities. How have you seen those conversations change? Are they different? Do you find yourself in a different dialogue with non-arts funders now than you did ten years ago? What are you seeing at the front edge of civic arts projects and the structures that support and sustain them?

Anne: Arts and health is a unique area. Liz Lerman talks so eloquently about the horizontal—about how all the art therapies (dance, theatre, poetry, visual art, etc.) can do amazing and very specific work with people with specific medical challenges. But artists who are not therapists also offer tremendous opportunities for improving general health conditions. I think we're seeing a moment in funding and practice where we are recognizing that those elements (artists in civic practice and art therapists) are not in competition but can complement each other quite effectively. Artists can ask questions and do things that inspire new ways of thinking about systems of care. Arts-based therapies, because of how they are funded and structured, tend to work within those systems.

The field of gerontology/aging has also seen enormous changes in its relationship to the arts. Just in the last ten years we've seen the formation and thriving of the National Center for Creative Aging and a flourishing of international groups focused on the same issue—bringing the arts to older adults as part of lifelong learning and general wellness. Countries that have national health systems tend to incorporate the arts as part of health prevention plans. In the United States, we've had to fight a little harder for the recognition that the arts are part of a healthy late life—even for those with significant cognitive and/or physical challenges. Because we over-medicalize aging in this country, the arts tend to be more associated with therapy. Are long-term care communities primarily health settings? Or are they simply communities where older people live — sometimes for decades? Long-term care communities could really benefit from all the amazing work that community-engaged social-practice artists are doing. In 2009, the Center on Age & Community at UWM convened a think tank about just that issue. We brought community-engaged artists who had never really worked in aging before into the same room with leading aging-services providers from around the country. It was great to have them learn, borrow, and build on each other's language.

So yes, I'm seeing lots of change. Arts funders are interested in the work. And social service / health funders are too. Even in the recession, which tends to push funders to take fewer risks, we were able to raise our entire budget for Penelope. I'm also really interested in what comes next. I'm hopeful that BA or BFA arts students can find a career path in "life enrichment" in care communities for older adults. I see it as another way to do both arts education and really innovative art-making simultaneously in a community setting that happens to provide health care. In some ways, this is part of Penelope's lasting impact — the project acts as a demonstration of the successful and valuable role of collaboration and co-creation among artists, students, and elders and their communities.

MAKING STRUCTURAL CHANGES IN THE CURRICULUM THROUGH PENELOPE
Robin Mello and Anne Basting

One of the lasting impacts of Penelope was a revisioning and overhaul of the UWM Department of Theatre's bachelor of arts curriculum. The Penelope engaged-learning course sequence enabled our colleagues to see clearly how such work could be embedded in the curriculum and become a powerful learning opportunity and viable career path for theatre students — and even draw new students to UWM and the department. To understand the magnitude of this change, we share a bit of the history of the program itself.

UWM's BA in theatre was first created in 2002 and included a small group of undergraduate courses with little cohesive curriculum except that students were required to take twenty-four credits in the major. Like many theatre BA programs across the country, ours struggles to maintain an identity and integrity in the shadow of the bachelor of fine arts programs in technical production and acting. The UWM Department of Theatre has a convergence of staff and faculty with interest and expertise in working in community-engaged theatre and strong local nonprofits in this area, including the Center for Applied Theatre and the Milwaukee Public Theatre. But we still had considerable work to do to explain what the Penelope classes and project could be — even in our own theatre department. When Sojourn was in residence in Milwaukee, we offered workshops for theatre students and invited them to join as guests at a department meeting. We invited national experts in theatre (Robbie Macauley, Elinor Fuchs) and in community-engaged performance in particular (Jan Cohen-Cruz, Lucy Winner, Pam Korza) to Milwaukee to hold a workshop (Using the Arts and Humanities in Community Health) as well as to see the final performance. This was an important element of legitimizing the work in the eyes of both students and faculty at our home institution.

The idea that Penelope could be a proving ground for BA programming was the underlying factor in our early decision to create Penelope Project courses. The resulting model — with its team approach to teaching, early and prolonged research and experimentation, service-learning experiences, development of performance through iterative and collaborative practices, and connecting with professional artists — is now an essential component of our BA curriculum. We've been replicating, revising, and experimenting with this model ever since.

After the *Finding Penelope* play closed in 2011, we created a proposal for overhauling the BA in theatre at UWM that built on the Penelope pilot structure, more fully integrated the theatre and education courses into the BA, and asserted the performative components of applied theatre courses. In the summer of 2012, Basting helped form the Creative Trust (www.creative trustmke.com), an alliance of care facilities and UWM Peck School of the Arts faculty and students committed to fostering lifelong learning through the arts. The Creative Trust would develop programming and provide on-going leadership and opportunities for intergenerational engagement in the arts. Each May, the Creative Trust holds the Flourish Festival, "a celebration of creativity as we age" that provides a showcase for intergenerational arts programming developed throughout the year.

In the new BA program, students enter as majors and take the core courses while also working on their university-to-degree credits (aka the general education requirements). Then, they engage in Storytelling, Participatory Theatre, a course on theatre education methods, and a choice of either Playwriting or Design and Communications. From there they take up to eighteen credits in theatre electives — using the department's offerings as a playground for exploration. Finally, students enroll in the community-based practice sequence: Performing Community and Performance Capstone. Performing Community orients them to the world of engaged theatre practice and gives them a chance to explore projects. Performance Capstone asks them to be part of a work-in-progress, to take on specific roles in that work, and to bring the work to fruition.

The changes in curriculum and the building of partnership infrastructures for the department have already yielded exciting results. In the fall of 2013, faculty member Alvaro Saar Rios directed and wrote a devised play called *Milwonky Style* that was built of stories about the UWM student experience. It was a great success for the department in terms of audience numbers and student enthusiasm, and *Milwonky II* was slotted for the 2014–2015 season. It too attracted a large student following, particularly among first- and second-year students. Robin Mello proposed an original, devised work — *Cinderella: The First 30,000 Years* — for the 2013–2014 season. Basting worked with the Creative Trust to offer three different community-engaged workshops to inform the content of *Cinderella*. The workshops were filmed and incorporated into the production itself as choreography, text, and media effects.

In 2014, Basting worked with the Creative Trust to hold intergenerational workshops inspired by the novel *Little Women*, including a letter exchange between Introduction to Women's Studies students and elders in the Creative Trust. In their letters, UWM students shared their dreams of their "castles in the air," as they call them in *Little Women*. The elders responded with advice and stories of their own dreams. In the spring semester of 2015, Basting worked with students to write and stage a performance dialogue called *Slightly Bigger Women*, inspired by the intergenerational and cross-cultural perspectives on the changes in women's lives since the novel's publication. It was designed as a "performance/dialogue," and elders from the Creative Trust and students from Introduction to Women's Studies attended to continue their conversation and to meet in person for the first time.

Basting and Maureen Towey reunited as co-lead artists on the Islands of Milwaukee, which was also offered as part of the new BA sequence. The project aimed to create a sustainable system for bringing creative engagement to older adults who are living alone or under-connected to their community. In spring 2013's Performing Community course, students became official volunteers for Interfaith Older Adult Programs, a local nonprofit providing support to older adults living at home. Working in pairs, students got to know several older adults by visiting them at home and coming up with creative ways to engage. That preliminary pilot work helped the Islands team create the "Questions of the Day" approach, in which simple questions are designed, printed, and distributed by volunteers as a way to engage the elders who are living alone or under-connected to their community. The responses are gathered by voicemail, handwritten on the cards themselves, or submitted via the project's website (islandsofmilwaukee.org).

In the fall of 2013, students in Storytelling used the Question of the Day system to engage with groups of older adults at Luther Manor and at the Jewish Home and Care Center in Milwaukee, culminating the semester with a "sharing" of the stories that emerged with both the UWM audience and an audience at the care facilities. In the spring of 2014, students who were selected by audition registered for Rehearsal and Performance and staged *The Crossings*—performances at crosswalks that area older adults have identified as too dangerous to cross. The goal of *The Crossings* was to train Milwaukee drivers to see and stop for pedestrians of any age. Students studied the traffic patterns of the intersections, helped create relationships with police and elders who live near the intersections, and devised and performed the street theatre. Civic officials were invited to attend each of the three *The Crossings*. We created special "public address" moments in which students shared the concerns of area elders and in which mayors, county supervisors, and state representatives could talk about what they planned to do about the issue.

Penelope's pilot three-course sequence has proven enormously fruitful for extended community-engaged projects. It allowed for long-term partnership development, meaningful community engagement, and a luxuriously long period for creative research. Students aren't required to take all three courses but instead have the flexibility to cycle in and out of a project based on their interests and the significant demands of their schedules. The intergenerational Creative Trust structure provides continuity of community partnerships beyond single projects and provides some regularity of structure for both the academic and the long-term care institutions. The rigorous evaluation of Penelope helped us make clear arguments for the impact on the students' learning experience, which helps garner additional resources and support for the work. Slowly, the department that had been founded as a professional theatre inside of a university was finding a home and appreciation for theatre that often spilled outside the walls of the theatre building itself.

WHAT DID THE RESEARCH TELL US?
Robin Mello and Julie Voigts

After the production of *Finding Penelope*, we analyzed the data we gathered from surveys; student field notes and reflections; interviews with artists, staff, and residents; and focus group transcripts from throughout the project. We looked at the data to determine the project's impact on all those involved: students, residents, staff, artists, and audience members. The program evaluation itself (available at thepenelopeproject.com) is nearly one hundred pages long. Here, we provide an excerpt from that longer report. Greater detail on the methodology of the program evaluation is provided in the appendix.

STUDENTS

UWM students participated in Penelope as learners, artists, crew, and researchers. To inform our evaluation of student engagement, we gathered and analyzed student reflections, discussion submissions, written essays, transcripts, action plans, questionnaires, and surveys.

A pre-survey designed to identify student perspectives and attitudes toward older adults prior to engaging in Penelope activities was administered at the start of the jointly offered Storytelling and Playwriting classes, before students went to Luther Manor. The same survey was administered again at the end of that fall 2010 semester and once again in April 2011 after the *Finding Penelope* play closed. Survey data suggest that the students' (whose median age was approximately nineteen years old) comfort, conceptions, and empathic perspectives were enhanced by their course work and service-learning experience.

Comparisons of pre- and post-survey (September and December) data suggest *significant* changes in attitudes (see table 2). Before participating in any Penelope activities the group was split between positive and neutral/negative ideas and dispositions toward the elderly. After Penelope activities, the majority of students surveyed said that they were more likely to visit an older relative, be comfortable around older adults, and were interested in assisting and supporting elders.

Notable change in attitudes can be seen in responses to these prompts: "I enjoy talking to old people," "I enjoy being around old people," and "I enjoy

TABLE 2. UWM STUDENT SURVEY RESULTS

Survey Question/Prompt	PRE-SURVEY (SEPT. 2010)			POST-SURVEY (DEC. 2010)		
	Disagree/ Strongly Disagree	Neutral	Agree/ Strongly Agree	Disagree/ Strongly Disagree	Neutral	Agree/ Strongly Agree
I enjoy being around old people	19%	24%	57%	14%	14%	72%
I like to go and visit my older relatives	19%	14%	67%	14%	14%	72%
I enjoy talking to old people	19%	5%	76%	0%	7%	93%
I feel very comfortable when I am around an old person	50%	37%	13%	7%	14%	79%
I enjoy doing things for old people	0%	33%	67%	0%	7%	93%
I believe that I'll still be able to do most things for myself when I am old	5%	14%	81%	14%	29%	57%
It is rewarding to work with people who have Alzheimer's disease or dementia	19%	57%	24%	14%	29%	57%
People with Alzheimer's disease or dementia can be creative	0%	31%	69%	0%	7%	93%

doing things for old people." In September, there was a range of responses. A little over half of students reported they enjoyed "being around old people." By December, just 14 percent of the students reported disliking these experiences, and the range of responses had also shrunk: 72 percent now liked being around older adults, and 93 percent enjoyed conversing with them.

Also significant are the responses to this prompt: "People with Alzheimer's disease or dementia can be creative." While none of the students (in pre- or post-surveys) disagreed with this statement, prior to engaging in Penelope course and service-learning work 31 percent were neutral. *After* Penelope, 93 percent strongly agreed that elders with dementia were able to create and engage in creative activities. Only 7 percent reported neutrality. These data indicate that the experience of creative engagement was an experience that supported a shift in students' dispositions toward elders.

Through our analysis of student assignments, we identified several key learning outcomes. Students made significant gains in their attitudes toward persons with dementia: they grew empathically and intellectually. Undergraduates also gained a deeper sense of being "part of a way bigger community" than they had previously. The course(s) also expanded their ideas of what theatre is and how it might be constructed. The site-specific nature of the work was almost revelatory to some. The ways that cast members improvised and developed material—iteratively and over long periods of experimentation—had a strong impact on students' perceptions of their own artistic skills and capabilities.

Most students felt that the course work was intellectually beneficial. They noted that they gained information and knowledge from the Penelope experience. Responses on questionnaires, in interviews, and to surveys included statements such as the following: "Amazing to work with the people at Luther Manor (LM). Hearing their stories changes my day and my thinking for the better," and "This has been an excellent experience. I think that every student [in this university] should be involved in a project like this at some time."

In the data, students expressed desire for UWM and the Department of Theatre to create more opportunities like this and to focus more course work on engaged, applied, and community oriented work: "I love the applied theatre that we are learning. I hope I can create similar ones in the future." A fairly typical response came from a sophomore who noted: "It is amazing being around these women [at my LM group], an enlightening experience. At first I was terrified. Now, it's funny to think I was. I want to do this again. Are there other courses like this?"

Students responded to Penelope course work by replicating the inclusive and caring models that they had been exposed to. When they were asked to take leadership roles in their interactive learning groups, they focused on ideas about interactive relationships, self-awareness, dignity, parity, and community. Comments included statements such as the following: "I am learning about the way I can now interact with the elders in our Milwaukee community," and "Now I've formed a deep respect and deep respected relationship with [my group]."

Discussing, considering, facing, and reflecting on death was a topic that kept cycling through the course discussions and reflections. One of the themes embedded in this student-generated data is the avoidance of the idea of death—a majority of undergraduates discussed being fearful of being near persons who were terminally ill and/or close to death. Most students entered the course with a strong sense of invincibility. They made the assumption that the young do not die young and that the old are both close to death and unable to engage in activities that the young enjoy (e.g., sexual intimacy, romantic love, innovative action, seeking adventure, contemporary music or media, etc.). They articulated naive or avoidance-oriented ideas about their own aging or about the elderly in their family or community.

This feeling may be why only 13 percent first reported feeling "comfortable" around old people (at the beginning of the academic year) yet were also optimistically oriented toward their own old age — a combination of fear and denial in action. By the end of the semester, this optimistic approach to their own end of life had shrunk from 81 percent to 57 percent. Also, their comfort in being around older adults increased. As the course proceeded, students' attitudes clearly shifted. Students discussed Penelope's story, shared their own perspectives, and actively listened to others' ideas and responses. This allowed them to develop a more nuanced, realistic, and practical impression of aging and dying — for example: "One of the things I keep thinking about is talking to Dr. Barr who died just after we talked to him! About sharing his memories of private airplanes," and "We tried to do something different every time so when we went to LM and lost a group member [who died] it was somehow OK."

The iterative nature of deeply community-engaged performance practice can leave students unsure of expectations and their own progress against them. Creating small, clear assignments that fit inside the iterative process can help offset that uncertainty and give students the clarity they need to feel successful in their creative explorations.

Students mentioned two other problems — ones that the Penelope leaders struggled over for some time: transportation and lack of mentoring (of students) during the devising period. The lack of reliable transportation, which haunts most community-engaged learning programs, was finally solved by Luther Manor, which generously offered free bus service to students in the fall and to students/actors in the spring.

THE STAFF AND RESIDENTS

[Being in Penelope] made me feel more alive. I was glad at the time
I got up and started coming to practice; I had stayed in bed too much.
And I got up and got involved. And I really enjoyed it. It helped me

*get along and involved. I had just gotten out of the hospital when I got
involved and it got me on my feet.*
—*LM Resident /* Finding Penelope *Chorus Member interview*

We analyzed field notes, interviews, and focus group transcripts to understand how residents participated in the project and what happened because
of that participation. We found that Luther Manor residents participated in
a wide range of Penelope activities, such as weaving, art-making, letter writing, and decorating Penelope's Room. They attended creative engagement
sessions facilitated by staff, students, and artists, and they attended rehearsals, performances, and postshow discussions all over the course of a year and
a half.

Interviews revealed that Luther Manor participants (both residents and
staff) viewed the creation of the play *Finding Penelope* as an innovative experience that filled their lives with interesting and unique challenges. Based
on the data, we identified several elements of the project that were particularly powerful for the residents. Luther Manor interviewees discussed the
quality of their Penelope experiences and appreciated the way they were encouraged to be *actively engaged* in the world of the play:

> What was special about it? I think what was special, between reading the
> book and the way you presented it—it's about strength and hope and
> love. And I have a lot of problems and I really feel each day is a blessing
> to me. And I think it showed that. And that all these people on the stage
> were Penelope. It was a beautiful ending. I think my favorite actor was
> her husband [Odysseus]. He just put himself right into it, I thought.
> When the welcome home, that one part, I thought I was going to cry.
> I didn't, but I came pretty close to it. . . . I shook hands with him and
> he came over a couple times before they closed it. It was nice. I really
> enjoyed being in it and being in something like that.
> —Resident / Chorus Member interview

> It helps you get out and get involved. . . . It really got me up and I went
> down there every day. I got up and got involved. I was a weaver. I liked
> doing it.
> —Resident / Chorus Member interview

Participants reported that they had "fun." They "enjoyed doing the play"
and liked it because it was "something different to do." One interviewee noted

that it engaged her creatively and intuitively: "I think the greatest thing that I learned was to continue to use my imagination and let my imagination fly." Another commented that being part of *Finding Penelope* made her feel useful: "It makes you feel that you're doing something, doing something for the public. You know."

> I don't think you want to lose the friendships you made with people in the play and watching the play and sitting and talking to people and hearing their comments and their ideas on the play. I think it was mostly very good 'cause it seemed like everybody enjoyed the play.
> — LM Resident / Chorus Member interview

Participants also recalled the themes embedded in the play and the plight of Penelope — as one member put it, "She had the courage!"

> That Penelope had patience. And all the idiots that wanted to marry her. I learned about Penelope when I was in grade school. And this was fun to think about these things all over again. Because that was a long time ago.
> — Resident / Chorus Member interview

> For a while she didn't seem to recognize him. He was gone for ten years and people change and everything changed. But in the end, they got together. *It's a happy ending.* Right. *Any other last words about it?* I think the thing that impressed me most of all is that we were all Penelope. It was in us.
> — Resident / Chorus Member interview

In interviews, two staff members reminded us that Penelope art-making had a profound effect on residents. They felt that one of the most crucial and important factors of the project was the way visual art was embedded into the creative explorations. They pointed out that residents and staff had opportunities to create nonrepresentational work inspired by Penelope's story. This abstract approach was significant to the project because it supported creative engagement and led to original and interesting responses. Penelope required participants to use abstract concepts, metaphors, creative dance, and expressive design in their explorations. For example, in the weaving sessions, fiber was provided, and questions were asked, such as, What color do you think Penelope *felt* like? Can you knit this material in a sad way?

In the focus group interview, held at the end of April 2011 after the play closed, key members of the "team," along with cast members and administrators, discussed their perspectives. All agreed that the experience had been positive, transformative, and/or profound.

> [Penelope is part of] Luther Manor culture [now], I think a lot of people saw it as just coming together as a spontaneous event, but I was aware of really how much your group kind of grappled, struggled, creatively, worked together. I think as a leader, I think we should all strive for that . . . and [acknowledge] those moments of spontaneity.
> — Administrator interview

They also remembered how confusing and overwhelming the program had been at first and how they began to see that confusion as productive.

> I think of it from the administrator in me: There were times when we would be meeting like this and we just didn't know how to do it. We would sit around here and [say], "How are we really gonna' get to the next step?" And I learned that we could do it. You know, I've worked here a long time. Most of us around this table have worked here a long time. We know that we do really good work here. And that you can work with another department and work together on a project and we could do it. I didn't know if we could do a project like this. We did it!
> — Administrator interview

Luther Manor staff and administration frequently defined their Penelope experience as a "challenge." They discussed the ways that the project had begun: "It was so challenging." They also used the word when discussing their recruitment of others: "We challenged folks to be part of this." One staff member noted, "At the beginning we didn't have any idea of what this was, and some of us were really confused. In fact, there are those who refused to do it."

> The word that comes to mind is challenge. Just watching everybody and trying to even explain the project and the concept. People were challenged just by that. People were challenged every single day. Whether or not they wanted to go to the program, if they wanted to be involved, if they wanted to embrace it or not. There are other words that kind of jump out from that. But challenge I think is the main word. Because so many folks were challenged.
> — Staff interview

But I think the transformation . . . that you're talking about, where folks were pushing against not being involved — and then all of a sudden for whatever reason they did get hooked and then we did see people coming over every day to be in the chorus and absolutely loving it.
— Staff interview

Staff and administration acknowledged that they experienced a great deal of discomfort while meeting the challenges brought by the project — and they noted that this dissonant experience allowed them to stretch: "That beginning discomfort. Not always easy. It stretched people, the institution, and all of us."

How did this shift in perspective, from initial discomfort and difficulty to a positive and inclusive experience, come about? Many staff felt that it was a combination of three things. First, key individuals advocated for the project and demonstrated a willingness to try things that might be new or uncomfortable. Second, the project itself was highly flexible. When concerns were voiced, changes were made to address issues as they emerged. Third, having UWM students work at the site during the fall of 2010 was deeply important: "It was the interaction between students and the residents. This interaction evolved and developed."

I was just thinking that my overall experience was, "Hooray for young people!" It felt good to be with young people again — no insult intended here — white hairs and all.
— Resident / Chorus Member interview

Working with UWM students in autumn paved the way for work with the actors in the winter/spring. Students had already visited, assisted, had meals, and participated in social events at Luther Manor before actors came and did the same. Student-facilitated activities and their culminating presentation at the end of the fall 2010 semester were important embedded endpoints. Having multiple stops along the way helped everyone value the project. It gave participants tangible outcomes that they could point to. Staff felt that these experiences were significant because Luther Manor had an opportunity to act as hosts and because they were unique and different from the norm; were unexpected and innovative; were inclusive; brought younger people into Luther Manor for significant periods of time; and gave residents a purpose.

And we've been talking about the experience, and one of them said you know as we get older . . . we don't feel like we're worth anything.

We kind of look at it and think nobody needs me; my kids don't need me; my parents are gone; my friends, some of them are gone. We all know that statistics show that people live longer when they feel that they are needed. . . . And here, these people felt needed. They needed to do the weaving; they needed to do the chorus. It was just a wonderful experience; it's been wonderful to share it as [a host] to have guests come into the facility.
— Staff interview

Luther Manor staff felt that another important component in the success of the project was being able to share and/or delegate the process to others. They referred to this as "letting go" (i.e., letting go of anxiety and worry, being responsible for success or failure, sharing ideas, letting someone else try something that you don't agree with, and flexing the institutional boundaries and control). As one administrator noted, "The minute I gave up on trying to control everything was when I started to really enjoy it."

I think that's a really good thing that we all learned to let go of the control. 'Cause in the beginning we were like, "Where's the schedule? Who is going to [do] it?" And then . . . the last three weeks we were like, "Just let me know when I'm supposed to show up!" [*General laughter.*] And [what] was really remarkable [was] to stand back and watch, that as we let go of the control, the residents and participants participated better.
— Staff interview

Another staff member agreed:

Yes! To just let it evolve, as it needed to evolve. And to stop trying to superimpose what we thought it should be or what we wanted it to be rather let it in the hands of those that were doing it. I think that the delight of the moment was something that I learned.
— Staff interview

The Penelope project spoke directly to the philosophical foundations of the institution and helped staff build connections across boundaries: "[What I don't want to lose] is the connections between people, the friendships I've made." Staff also learned to value the meetings and planning sessions and emphasized the significance of the face-to-face engagement that Penelope activities required.

The theme that was developed, about faith, waiting, being separated from a loved one, the joy of reunion: I don't know if you came in with that idea or if it arose from your meeting and seeing what happens here at Luther Manor, but I thought that was just right on. And from what I'd seen, portrayed beautifully.

— Administrator interview

Staff and administrators acknowledged that the longer they were involved with the project, the more they valued it. It became an excellent example of the "Seven Values" articulated by Luther Manor's Adult Day Services, Luther Manor's overall mission, and the tenets of person-centered care. Penelope embodied and personified person-centered care in its community perspective, inclusive vision, and use of celebration. This made a significant impact on residents and staff alike. As one staff observed: "In the end, it is the sharing, hospitality, and gathering of community that really counted. Since the biggest challenge here (on my unit) is long-term memory, the idea of celebration was easiest to grasp. But the Penelope Project also created connections to the volunteers and myself. I discovered that we are family."

THE ARTISTS

One of the more unique aspects of the Penelope Project was its impact and effect on the professional artists who came to Luther Manor to work on it. Some Sojourn Theatre members were recruited because they had professional experience working in therapeutic, educational, or long-term care facilities. All of these artists came prepared and interested in meeting the goals of the project, with deep experience in community engagement.

An analysis of the group interviews, field notes, and pre- and post-survey data shows that at the beginning of the devising and rehearsal process, most Sojourn company members were already comfortable with the idea of working around elders (see table 3), but some expressed uncertainty regarding how to work efficiently with persons with dementia.

Company members experienced a modest, yet highly significant, shift in perspective during their work on *Finding Penelope*. A pivotal moment took place during the rehearsal process. Cast members had their first encounter with a resident's death. This is a common occurrence at Luther Manor, and staff members expect to encounter the dying during their daily work routine. They are trained to follow protocols designed to manage interactions with

TABLE 3. ARTIST SURVEY RESULTS

Survey Question/Prompt	PRE-SURVEY (JAN. 2011)			POST-SURVEY (APR. 2011)		
	Neutral[1]	Agree	Strongly Agree	Neutral	Agree	Strongly Agree
I enjoy being around old people	25%	75%	0%	0%	67%	33%
I like to go visit my older relatives	25%	50%	25%	0%	67%	33%
I enjoy talking to old people	0%	75%	25%	0%	67%	33%
I feel very comfortable when I am around an old person	50%	50%	0%	33%	67%	0%
I enjoy doing things for old people	25%	75%	0%	0%	100%	0%
I believe that I'll still be able to do most things for myself when I am old	25%	50%	25%	67%	33%	0%
It is rewarding to work with people who have Alzheimer's disease or dementia	25%	75%	0%	0%	33%	67%
People with Alzheimer's disease or dementia can be creative	0%	50%	50%	0%	33%	67%

Notes

1. No artists responding to these surveys ever chose "Disagree" or "Strongly Disagree." Standard deviations of these data ranged from .00 to .58.

the dead, family members, and the medical community. For actors, however, this was not a standard experience.

The company members were unsettled yet responded in a professional and caring manner. They discussed the event and took time for reflection. They approached administrators and activities directors for advice and feedback. When rehearsals resumed, they did so with a slightly more serious quality. The experience added resonance to the production and also served to deepen the artists' connection to the themes within the play and overall goals of the project.

After completing the play, the Sojourn artists expressed nuanced views of their relationship with their own aging and focused much of their discussion (in interviews and focus groups) on the meaningful interactions with persons with dementia. Survey data show a shift from "neither agree nor disagree" toward "agreement," especially in areas of "comfort" around elders, enjoyment while "talking to old people," and "doing things for" elderly persons.

Like the audience members, a majority of artists found that the tensions and problematic conditions addressed by the play *Finding Penelope* (loss of dignity, searching for meaning at the end of life, warehousing and devaluing of elders, etc.) were amplified by the experience of making the piece. At the end of the experience, no one remained neutral and 33 percent now strongly agreed with the statement "I enjoy being around old people." Overall, data indicated that actors' perspectives on aging expanded while their understanding of the potential of elders and elders' status/value was reinforced. Clearly, Penelope was a deeply meaningful experience for artists.

THE AUDIENCE

> *The play really affected me. . . . I was moved to tears by the closing scene, being reminded that elderly residents are incredibly unique and gifted, and have made tremendous contributions to society in their lifetime. This performance encouraged me to look deeper [at the elders I meet].*
> —*Audience survey*

Approximately two hundred official, ticketed audience members experienced the play *Finding Penelope* during previews and productions. As many as two hundred more were "unofficial" audience members—residents, staff, family, and students who came to observe the play as it moved through Luther Manor. Audience members who provided contact information through ticket sales were emailed one month after the play closed. In an online, anonymous survey, attendees were asked to respond to a series of prompts, choice questions, and short-answer queries. The response rate was approximately 32 percent of all ticketed audience members.

The survey asked for written comments about powerful moments in the play. Many audience members focused on *Finding Penelope*'s family/community connection. A smaller, but significant, minority chose to reflect on the artistic vision, quality, and construction of the work—spotlighting the collaborative and/or creative nature of the play (rather than its community impact). These two different perspectives sometimes led to dissimilar attitudes and ideas about the quality, intent, effect, and purpose of the production.

All audience respondents thought that *Finding Penelope* was a "meaningful experience"; 95 percent agreed that it "taught them something"; and 84 percent commented that it was unique and also inclusive. Moreover, 74 percent of survey respondents said, "It was entertaining," and 14 percent saw the play as an "opportunity." There were no divergent data trends in this section of the survey. All audience members who chose to answer survey questions were positively oriented to the production; *Finding Penelope* was a meaningful, educational, surprising, and/or unique theatrical experience.

When audience members were asked what surprised them about *Finding Penelope*, most reported being amazed by the many ways that the play included Luther Manor residents: "The involvement of the residents, it was so cool! They welcomed us in their midst, in their home." Most had expected to see a play that was "realistic," and they went away astonished by the site-specific nature of the work, the "flowing nature" of the production, and how "logistics" were executed in such a "smooth and seamless" fashion. Other surprises were the amount of humor embedded in the show, its "cleverness," and the forceful emotional content.

A majority of audience members responded to our survey by describing the play as a deeply affecting and moving experience. They reported "reliving" the play in their minds well after it was over and also connecting it to their own lives. Remembering the play prompted audience members to share their own memories of aging, love, and loss. In effect, they "discovered" Penelope — either by recalling powerful connections that they (or their loved ones) had with Penelope's plight or by identifying with "being Penelope."

> Overall, I can relive just about every single "act." It continued to grow and grow and grow until, at the very end, when Penelope was with her daughter and the two of them were conversing I found myself slowly melting with emotion. THEN, THE CURTAINS OPENED. I was absolutely an emotional mess. I was awestruck at how the "actors" on stage oh-so-carefully watched the leader (sitting down center stage), and mimicked all of her actions. So innocent. So engaged. (At this point, as tears streamed down my face, I wondered why in the world I would have chosen to take a front row seat!) My own mom died two years ago, suddenly, without warning. I wished so, so much that she could have been on stage . . . or, knowing my mom, she would have been Penelope!
> — Audience survey

> There were moments that really touched me, like when they started tearing out the weaving and reciting the women's life stories backward.

And when Odysseus fights Alzheimer's and looks so lost and confused. That look was exactly how my grandmother looked sometimes. She died of Alzheimer's in 2008. Thank you for making this project.
— Audience survey

Approximately 57 percent of audience members identified the *Odyssey* and/or "the myth of Penelope" when recalling and discussing the show.

I like that it celebrated the mythic and the fantastic, as well as the very ordinary middle-class lives of the everyday and the beauty and struggle within each of them.
— Audience survey

I loved the intertwining of myth and contemporary reality: the theme of "home," the search for a loved one, and all the fears that can surround that quest [were] beautifully realized. The symbolism of the weaving, the suit coats for the suitors, the actual traveling throughout the building, the "chorus" of Luther Manor residents all contributed to a delightful juxtaposition of reality and metaphor and definitely contributed to a feeling of warmth toward the "home" that Luther Manor has become for so many people.
— Audience survey

A number of audience members also noted that the play was not easy to experience: "It was unsettling," and "There were many painful moments." Emotional responses included grief, regret, anger, and guilt. This reaction seemed to deepen and intensify the "meaningful nature and experience of seeing the play." It also made it difficult to watch.

Generally, American contemporary society tends to equate positive and optimistic emotions with positive outcomes. However, this data challenges that assumption. Audience members made direct associations between despair and hope, joy and sorrow, angst and clarity. They found this dialectic stressful but meaningful. The message of the play was communicated through these emotional states powerfully and persuasively.

The fact that I was personally moved to tears. It flooded me with memories of my mother who did not live long enough to reach a nursing home. It hit a cord with me and my unnamed fear of growing old. It gave me hope.
— Audience survey

While [it] was unsettling I also felt that it was very powerful to move through the space because so much of what I saw, smelled and experienced added layers to the production that I would have never gotten if I had watched this piece on a stage.
— Audience survey

The layers of meaning and the way I arrived at my feelings about how we treat/ignore our elderly . . . how we shut them away . . . how we make them useless by excluding them . . . all of that was deepened and integrated because of the way the piece was delivered. So I had a complicated reaction, which I think is evidence of a complex and profound piece of art.
— Audience survey

Spectators praised and appreciated the professional and site-specific nature of the piece, commenting on how it moved through Luther Manor and praising the fact that at each of the five scene locations there were different members of the community interwoven into the performance. Others appreciated the structure of the play's performance in relation to written text, its resonance, and the "dramatic use" of true stories and perspectives. In one instance, a respondent craved information about the consenting process in order to clarify her responsibility as an audience member and mitigate the uncomfortable feeling of having walked through someone's home while not aware of whether she was truly welcomed.

What was most dynamic about the experience was moving through the center and the blurred line it created of who was watching whom.
— Audience survey

THE ESSENTIAL ELEMENTS OF PENELOPE
Robin Mello and Julie Voigts

After analyzing all project data, we identified seven elements that contributed to the positive outcomes of the Penelope Project. We break each element into several characteristics.

ELEMENT #1: EXTENDED AND PROGRESSIVE EVOLUTION

The Penelope Project took place over more than three years. It was an extended and multifaceted endeavor that involved a significant number of people, funding organizations, sponsors, and others representing diverse institutions and viewpoints.

Multiple funding sources and flexible sponsorship

Multiple and diverse perspectives represented by the funding organizations enhanced the program's stated mission by broadening the audience base; modeling partnership across cultural, medical, and educational communities; and widening the possible impact at the local, national, and international levels.

Multiple endpoints and opportunities for feedback

Momentum was sustained over time by the project's numerous end points that acted as an external reward system. The most significant end points were the Storytelling students' presentations (December 2010) and the play itself (March 2011). But smaller end points included the creation of Penelope's Room/gallery, the creation of the educational guide, the completion of the weaving, and nearly every other creative activity related to the Penelope theme that had a tangible outcome. These all encouraged additional investment of time, resources, and ideas and gave participants concrete evidence of what was happening. Participants learned to focus on the small products, and this helped alleviate concerns about the viability and success of the final product(s).

Maintaining respect, acknowledgment, and
acceptance of input from diverse perspectives
From the very beginning, a functional and respectful tone was established by core participants. Input was welcomed and treated with respect. A great deal of the decision-making was done by consensus.

Plasticity and high tolerance for change
The plasticity of the project was a direct result of the committed and intense work that all participants put into the project. Leaders did their homework with more than due diligence. Simplistic as it seems, reading the *Odyssey* at the start of the project also added to the project's success.

Extending invitations and including participants over time
One of Penelope's strengths lay in its partnerships. Paradoxically, one of its biggest challenges was finding buy-in and coordinating institutional efforts. At times one institutional partner would move quickly while another was just getting up to speed. This demanded extra care with communications among the partnership network.

Welcoming the use of expertise and modeling an open-door policy
The project focused its energies first on those individuals who were interested in participating. With patience, the project then encouraged the input of naysayers, reticent staff, and others who were confused or cautious. It did so by modeling outcomes, keeping in contact, and hosting meetings. The project's open-door policy welcomed and shared information with anyone interested in the project. Hospitality grew to be an essential role in the overall success of the project.

Progression toward a high-impact outcome
The project built toward a culminating event (the play) that created a sense of pride within the community and that expanded the community (through audience). The high stakes and public outcome served to support the goals of the project.

ELEMENT #2: DEVISING AND CREATIVE PRACTICE
The project's identity evolved through a process of joint creation, experimentation, and devised (collaborative) theatre making.

Focusing on participants' expertise, interests, and needs
Penelope activities were designed to meet the needs of the constituents from each partnering institution, reflecting person-centered care practices.

Building agreement through devising
Negotiating expectations of what the play could or should support and what the final production would look like took a great deal of experimentation, discussion, and diplomacy. Ultimately this process gave partners a chance to take ownership while sharing the risk.

Using staff and contributor expertise
In addition to outside expertise, Penelope featured in-house staff members, teachers, and residents' expertise. Acknowledging the interdisciplinary expertise of participants strengthened the project—making it more efficient, less prescriptive, and directly connected to participants' lives.

ELEMENT #3: INTEGRATION AND ACCEPTANCE
Penelope provided opportunities for persons in long-term care to have and demonstrate that they could meet high expectations with success. It directly challenged the stigmatization of people with cognitive or physical disabilities. The project was able to address oppressive themes and conditions—such as ageism, fear of death, and sexism—in informed and pragmatic ways.

Integration and acceptance as a value system
The person-centered care value system (the assurance of individuality, choice, privacy, dignity, respect, independence, and a sense of being, to create home) was established practice at Luther Manor's Adult Day Center. A similar set of values had developed at Sojourn Theatre during the past twelve years. Blending these value systems inside the project supported its success.

Integration and acceptance as curriculum
The tenets and perspectives of Penelope also became part of the curriculum for participating UWM students.

Integration as practice
Penelope demonstrated the strength of collaborative teamwork. At UWM, team-teaching was seminal to the impact the project had on student learn-

ing. At Luther Manor, staff from multiple areas began to work in concert — the shift in culture at Luther Manor occurred not only because it was inclusive but also because Penelope required that staff and residents come out of isolation.

Fighting assumptions
Penelope helped destigmatize persons with disabilities and the elderly by bringing people out of isolation and casting them in the production. It also challenged stereotypes of women by calling attention to the power of waiting, homemaking, crafting, and caretaking. It gave residents a sense of purpose and stimulated their interest and imagination. Students' and artists' perceptions of aging and disability changed positively.

Fighting stigma and fear
Data also show that the project followed through on its promise to model caring and ethical perspectives. Some of the final architectural decisions of *Finding Penelope* — such as placing scenes and rehearsals in the Health Care Center, Faith and Education Center, Courtyards, Welcome Center, hallways, dining areas, and residents' rooms — required greater cooperation between staff, artists, and families. This led to a sense of team building and collaboration, which in turn led to a gradual easing of some stigma and fear pertaining to death, infirmity, and dementia.

Public and private (secular/nonsecular) collaborations necessitated tolerance and acceptance of differing beliefs and approaches
One of the most unique characteristics of Penelope was its ability to support an ethical framework that incorporated and respected the diversity of participants. The project balanced the needs and standards supported by its public secular partners (UWM and Sojourn Theatre) and Luther Manor (a private institution that is in partnership with the Evangelical Lutheran Church in America and the Greater Milwaukee Synod).

ELEMENT #4: APPLYING MYTH
Penelope explored the *Odyssey*, a 2,700-year-old story that offers important archetypal and universal information about the human condition. By examining the archetypes of Odysseus and Penelope, the project created a shared metaphoric language.

Identifying common purposes
The one constant of the project was Penelope's story—her struggles, obstacles, perspective, and fate. Exploring Penelope's dilemmas provided an empathic connection across institutions, groups, activities, and outcomes.

Establishing mythic conversation
Using the *Odyssey* provided participants with an opportunity to explore mythic symbols, a time-honored tool for encouraging conversations about beliefs and personal vision.

Using myth to promote creative engagement
Penelope made use of mythic time in order to encourage creative engagement. Mythic time allowed individuals freedom to use imagination and identify directly with the powerful images and information embedded in Homer's text.

Honoring and including the spiritual framework of all participants
The ethical and spiritual systems discussed in the *Odyssey* were used to acknowledge universal questions such as life and death, love and loss, grief and guilt. The *Odyssey* not only provided a typology that could be applied to psychological and interpersonal interactions; it also gave participants a way to explore compassion and ethics. The fact that the play focused on an ancient saga that was not bound up in any contemporary dogma or system of belief allowed collaborators to explore their own convictions more freely.

ELEMENT #5: CO-PARTNERING AND
BUILDING INTERGENERATIONAL AND
INTERINSTITUTIONAL COMMUNITY
Partnering was an essential component to both the evolution and growth of the program. Intergenerational partnerships made the project even stronger. The old learned and benefited from the young and vice versa.

Partnering as a developmental experience
Although partnering was built into the original concept, it soon became part of the way the project moved and evolved, and adding partners created new avenues for experimentation.

Partnering for artistic integrity
Partnering also allowed the project to design spaces and presentations so that they were accessible and artistically viable. Relying on the expertise of qualified professionals who worked in concert provided the project with choices and alternatives that supported the project's success.

Full participation from all partners
Having enough partners to shoulder the immense workload and diverse needs of constituents made it possible for the project to endure. Core groups began to be called "teams." The UWM students were a team, as were the staff/activities directors at Luther Manor. Eventually, this language evolved to include anyone involved in Penelope. Being part of a team made participants feel that they belonged to something larger than themselves.

Teams assumed specific roles and jobs
Separate teams took various roles and jobs. As the project learned to delegate and let go of micromanagement, it also came to rely on each team to follow through. Instead of duplicating efforts, time and expertise was used more efficiently.

ELEMENT #6: RIGOR
Project leaders shared an understanding that professional standards and competencies were essential values. They felt that high expectations for educational, care, and artistic practices were essential.

Linking conscientious practices together
Collaborators came to the project with highly developed aesthetic perspectives and beliefs. Sojourn Theatre, for example, has built its reputation by focusing on rigorous attention to specific devising processes, ensemble work, and theatrical craft. Luther Manor has long developed and refined its "Seven Values," implementing them in strict and formal ways. Anne Basting has created the nationally recognized program TimeSlips by carefully honing improvisational storytelling practices and combining it with best practices in dementia care and artistic practices. Robin Mello has been infusing her teaching and program curricula with contemporary and best practices connected with international and national standards and frameworks. These perspectives brought a deep understanding of, respect for, and commitment to engage in careful and meticulous processes and outcomes.

Devising contemporary models of theatre
Devising theatre in a given site is a very specific theatre practice that is under-going a renaissance within contemporary American theatre. *Finding Penelope* advanced our methodological knowledge by building live performance on the rhythms and structures of everyday life at Luther Manor. This in turn had an impact on audiences. After experiencing *Finding Penelope*, audience members — especially those unfamiliar with site-specific collaborative perfor-mance work — were moved, were engaged, had meaningful experiences, and felt welcomed to the space.

ELEMENT #7: CO-INSPIRED/CO-CREATED
The project leaders were inspired by each other. They allowed each other to shape processes through advising and adding, altering, and subtracting de-tails and ideas as needed.

Partnering
Each institution participated by doing what it did well. However, each insti-tution was also flexible and took on new ideas or perspectives. The project helped its institutions to thrive.

Il parenti
Each partner began from a place of expertise, adding and evolving additional perspectives over time and as individuals became more deeply involved. It was this critical involvement (combined with a respectful approach to sharing and listening to the expertise of others) that created an ultimate sense of be-longing to something important. This approach made the site-specific play *Finding Penelope* possible. Here audience members found themselves wel-comed into a performance event that was inclusive and interpersonally sig-nificant.

There is a word in Italian, *parenti*, a false cognate, that is often mistrans-lated in English as "parents of" or "relation to." It actually means the group of people who are connected to someone by custom, love, or friendship. One's *parenti* are one's tribe or honorary family. In the case of Penelope a majority of participants became *parenti*. The project generated a sense of belonging. Penelope built community even as it illustrated and gave voice to one.

THE LANDSCAPE BEYOND PENELOPE
Anne Basting, Ellie Rose, and Maureen Towey

The program evaluation team was incredibly thorough in teasing out what happened in the many phases of Penelope and in articulating the characteristics that contributed to the project's success. Penelope worked. It created an enriched environment of possibility and growth. It was meaningful for nearly everyone involved. For the duration of the project at least, the care community—which by regulation and mission strives to reduce risk—opened itself to creativity, collaboration, unprecedented changes in routine, and opening its doors to outsiders. The artists expanded their skills in partnership with people with profound disabilities. The students stepped into a landscape that provided context to their lives.

As artists, as scholars, as care providers, and—perhaps most importantly—as people aging ourselves, we now find ourselves driven to make normal this experience of meaningful, intergenerational connection and growth. We long for Penelope to be unexceptional. How does the landscape have to change to make this work unexceptional? In this essay, we look back to the first section and address the landscapes of university education, of the arts, and of long-term care to call out changes that we see beginning to stir. And we encourage that stirring in the hopes that more and more Penelopes will emerge.

Arts and humanities training at colleges and universities should integrate service learning into their core courses. The exploration of the human condition through literature, history, language, music, performance, and visual art is made richer by sharing that exploration with others. Co-learning in community settings now has strong research to suggest that it brings home concepts more than studying from books alone or than individual practice in a studio. New trends in "social innovation" in higher education have the potential to expand on this base of service learning to encourage arts and humanities students to create their own programs to engage and change the way social services are offered. At UWM, we are creating a pipeline from service learning to social innovation through our Student Startup Challenge programming. Students are hungry to know: How do you create a business model for a social innovation? How do you identify markets? How do you build the confidence to talk with a CEO of a care community and clearly articulate your assets as an artist? Students should have guidance to bring the deep learning born of engaged classroom experiences all the way through to the nonprofit (and for-profit) social service marketplace. Integrating the arts and humanities into long-term care isn't just a feel-good moment in a given class. It can shape an entire education. It can shape a life. It can provide a living.

To get there, long-term care and community-based care agencies need to consider students with applied arts and public humanities training for positions. Theatre BA student and Penelope participant Julie Voigts was hired at Luther Manor after demonstrating her significant skills in person-centered care and engagement. Life enrichment specialist is the new name for what used to be called activity director. These positions commonly no longer demand activity director certification but rather ask for a BA and field experience. Silverado, a forward-thinking long-term care community, has a "director of community engagement." Luther Manor staff member and arts-trained Ellie Rose recently completed Leading Age's year-long Leadership Academy alongside CEOs and COOs. As these positions in long-term care continue to change, and as the skill sets of students in the arts and humanities are expanded and deepened, the two should meet to create new career opportunities. This has great potential to radically alter the face of long-term care.

For Penelope to become normal, we need to accept the marriage of rigorous art-making and rigorous community engagement. There is no need to assume art made in deep and thorough community partnership is somehow "less than" art hanging in the museum or playing on equity stages. With the growth of social practice in the arts and in civic performance in theatre (see Michael Rohd's essay in part one), we are heading in this direction. We just need to keep walking this walk. Funding organizations (NEA, ArtPlace, Surdna, etc.) that have supported this shift need to continue their efforts or the trend will lose its strong footing. More funding partners can enter the space by expanding their existing areas of support (such as children's health or environmental issues) to include the rigorous engagement of arts partners in these areas.

To further develop social/civic practice in the arts as fields, the arts marketplace needs to figure out how to tell the story of this deeply partnered work and how to value it and reward the artists. Journalists and critics writing about this work still tell the story of the individual artist as genius who inspires a community to transform. One need only to read the stories of Theaster Gates, Paul Chan, and Candy Chang to understand the difficulty of telling these stories in a way that mirrors the complexity of the relationships and contexts from which they emerge. Should artists create collectives out of deeply partnered community projects? How can new creative models of licensing help this field become financially viable for artists and community partners alike? We don't have the answers, or even all the questions. But the mythology of individual artist as genius (and individual copyright holder ...) will need to change as this field grows.

For projects and partnerships like Penelope to become normal in long-term care, they must be accepted as part of the workload of all staff—from maintenance to certified nursing assistants to clinical nursing staff to administrators. If an environment is to become a place of meaning, meaningful expression must be invited from all community members. The skills of the "outside" artist partner include how to engage a community in dialogue, how to reflect that community back to itself, and how to invite expression that presents opportunities for growth, change, and connection. Those skills should be embraced and paid for by CEOs in care communities, just as they would myriad other consultants brought on to improve their businesses.

Meaningful engagement is currently the purview of the activity staff. But activities are at best two to three hours during each day. Is that the duration of meaningfulness for residents? For staff? For visitors? Meaningfulness needs to be poured into the daily life of care communities so that expression and the opportunity to contribute to a larger project can be part of every exchange. Conversations could flower while a staff member walks someone to a physical therapy appointment. Moments such as bathing, brushing teeth, staring out the window, sharing a meal—all these can become infused with meaning. There is no reason to turn off the invitation for meaningfulness. Art and creativity is more than paintbrushes and musical instruments. It is more than entertainment and distraction. Art-making gives us a way of being in relationships. It can invite us into recognizing and being present with each other. It can connect us across disability, culture, and generation. As artists, as teachers, as learners, as human beings on the journey to old age ourselves, this is all that we can hope for.

APPENDIX 1

PENELOPE PROJECT TIMELINE

PHASE 1	PLANNING AND RESEARCHING
Winter 2009	Preplanning with major collaborators
Spring 2010	Student seminar for dramaturgical research
	Sojourn and research team present at NAAP conference
	Sojourn and research team present at LM
	Sojourn artist residency: first visit
	Evaluation activities begin
Summer 2010	LM staff begin recruiting participation and planning activities
	Working with classicist Andrew Porter
	Course development
	IRB request submitted and approved

PHASE 2	PROGRAMMING AND TEACHING
Fall 2010	LM staff implement activities and begin formalizing plans to support students
	Sojourn workshop and auditions for *Finding Penelope* at UWM
	Artist residency with Sojourn at LM (1 week in October)
	Course delivery at UWM and LM
	Artist and collaborator visits and presentations at LM
	Evaluation data begun
	Documentary begins
December 2010	Public celebration of student work at LM
January 2011	Sojourn residency for devising and ensemble work at LM (1 week)

PHASE 3	PERFORMING
February 2011	Rewriting and production with Sojourn Theatre and Anne Basting
March 2011	4-week Sojourn residency
	Rehearsal and performance at LM

PHASE 4	MODELING/DISSEMINATION
April 2011	Think tank at UWM
	Post-production follow-up
	Interviews and surveys of participants and audience
Summer 2011	Evaluation report begins
	Presentations made at national and regional conferences
	Preplanning for summer institute
	Beyond Penelope begins at LM
	Raw footage of documentary complete

Fall/Winter 2011	Presentations made at national and regional conferences
Spring 2012	*Create/Change* Summer Institute
	Book proposal and book group formed
Summer 2012	Book group meets
	Evaluation report submitted
	Documentary in process

APPENDIX 2. PENELOPE PROJECT TEAM (IN ALPHABETICAL ORDER)

PENELOPE PROJECT LEADERS

Anne Basting: Director of UWM's Center on Age & Community (formerly); Associate Professor of Theatre at UWM; Project Director of Penelope; Writer of *Finding Penelope*; Instructor of Playwriting and Performance Workshop courses (fall 2010 / spring 2011); Codirector of *Create/Change* Summer Institute.

Robin Mello: Director of Theatre Education at UWM Department of Theatre; Area Head of BA Theatre Studies; Associate Professor of Theatre, Instructor of Storytelling course (fall 2010); Lead Evaluator for Penelope Project; Actor (old nurse).

Beth Meyer-Arnold: Director of Adult Day Services at Luther Manor; Lead Luther Manor Representative; Executive Committee Member of UWM's Center on Age & Community; Codirector of *Create/Change* Summer Institute.

Michael Rohd: Founder and Artistic Director of the Sojourn Theatre; Assistant Professor of Theatre at Northwestern University.

Maureen Towey: Ensemble Member of Sojourn Theatre; Director of *Finding Penelope*; Workshop Leader and Developer of *Create/Change* Summer Institute.

LUTHER MANOR SUPPORT TEAM

Lead Staff

Kathi Brueggemann, Resource Manager, Terrace

Tom Christopher, Director of Security

Nancy Kriske, Life Enrichment, Terrace

Linda Moscicki, Social Worker, Terrace

Mark Mrozek, Life Enrichment, Courtyards; Musical Arranger for *Finding Penelope*

Mark Powers, Life Enrichment, Health Care Center; *Finding Penelope* Musician

Ellie Rose, Manager and Person-Centered Care Specialist, Adult Day Services

Jean Tillmann, Life Enrichment, Health Care Center; Actor in *Finding Penelope*

Luther Manor Support Team Members

Terri Bartlett, Activity Director, Health Care Center

David Beinlich, Director of Health Care Center

Rebecca Chipman, Public Relations

Jolene Hansen, Volunteer, Adult Day Center

Kristy Johnson-Fofanah, Client Relations, Courtyards

David Keller, CEO of Luther Manor

Linda Lueck, Congregational Relations

Amy Quartaroli, Social Worker, Health Care Center
Jennifer Rust-Keefe, Social Work Intern, Adult Day Center
Cheryl Schmitz, Director of Volunteers
Ericka Tole, Director of Information Technology

SOJOURN THEATRE CORE TEAM
Daniel Cohen, Performer
James Hart, Performer
Rebecca Martinez, Performer
Michael Rohd, Artistic Director
Shannon Scrofano, Designer
Maureen Towey, Director
Nikki Zaleski, Performer

APPENDIX 3. PARTNERSHIP AGREEMENT

UWM DEPARTMENT OF THEATRE ROLES/EXPECTATIONS

(1) Students will enroll in a class (Storytelling or Playwriting) for the fall semester and participate in sharing and shaping stories about the themes in Penelope.

(2) Student Assistant Director to work with Sojourn Director Maureen Towey.

(3) Student Assistant Stage Manager to work with Sojourn Stage Manager.

(4) Student team can assist Sojourn multimedia artist on sound, video, web components.

(5) Student writers can assist Basting and Towey in the shaping of the script over Winterim.

(6) Student performers (likely three or four) can work with Sojourn performers and residents/staff/family in the shaping, rehearsal, and performance in spring 2010. This can be arranged for credit.

(7) Students in management and/or theatre education can work on the producing of the project (including creation of support materials) with Basting for credit.

(8) Students in theatre education and general BA can work with Robin Mello and Basting on the development of curricular materials from the project in year two.

(9) Sojourn can hold a workshop on "Outreach" for all theatre students (current and former) during their residency.

(10) Basting will apply for funds to support students to work with her in the run-up to the project — doing research, grant writing, communication, and relationship building.

(11) Basting will include percentages of her time, Mello's time, and the time of others supporting the project in grant proposals. We will also include supply/production costs in grant proposals.

(12) Any revenue from curricular materials will be shared equitably with UWM's CAC and Department of Theatre.

LUTHER MANOR ROLES/EXPECTATIONS

(1) Staff, volunteers, family, residents, and participants can choose to participate in discussions about the myth of Penelope and to be part of the creation and/or performance of a play.

(2) Participating staff will be trained in person-centered care along with their co-collaborators from UWM and Sojourn Theatre.

(3)   LM participants can be part of the discussions to shape curricular materials for general, professional, and academic audiences.

(4)   Any revenue from curricular materials will be shared equitably with LM.

(5)   Grants will ask for partial support for a LM-based project coordinator.

(6)   LM staff will assist in the writing of grants to support the project.

SOJOURN THEATRE ROLES/EXPECTATIONS

(1)   Grant proposals will request support for two weeks of a Sojourn residency in the fall of 2010, and six weeks in the spring of 2011. Sojourn members will also be consultants on the design and creation of curricular materials. Travel, lodging, and per diem costs will be included in grant proposals.

(2)   Participating Sojourn members will take the person-centered care training at LM with students and LM staff.

(3)   Sojourn members will potentially oversee student assistants during the project.

(4)   Sojourn members will offer a workshop to the Department of Theatre and community (those not involved in the project) during their residency.

(5)   Any revenue from curricular materials will be shared equitably with Sojourn.

(6)   Sojourn will assist in the writing of grants to support the project.

PARTNERSHIP GUIDELINES

(1)   Sojourn Theatre, UWM's Center on Age & Community, UWM's Department of Theatre, and Luther Manor are the core collaborative partners in this project.

(2)   Each core collaborative partner will identify members to serve on the collaborative team.

(3)   The collaborative team members will participate in regular planning and production meetings. All decisions about the shape of the project will be made by the collaborative team.

(4)   All revenues will be shared equitably by the core collaborative partners.

(5)   All core collaborative partners will have rights to use products of the project in promotion and educational presentations.

(6)   No changes can be made to the products of the project without approval of current representatives of the core collaborative partners.

APPENDIX 4. PROMPTS FOR PENELOPE ACTIVITIES AND CHALLENGES

As the artists, students, and Luther Manor staff and volunteers explored Penelope with family and residents, we created a series of activities to invite interpretation of the epic story. Sometimes we invited people to try something we genuinely didn't know how to accomplish. We called these "challenges." Throughout the creative discovery phase of the project, the staff grew more accustomed to saying yes to challenges and tackling them without any direction. We share this list of activities and challenges here to give readers an idea of the breadth of artistic lenses we used in the project and of the sheer amount of creativity that was transforming the Luther Manor environment.

(1) Zeus gave Penelope the gift of endurance. What is the greatest gift you've been given? Make a physical symbol of that gift.

(2) What is a "hero's journey"?

    (a) Whom do you consider a hero in your everyday life? Why? Does this person know that he or she is a hero?

    (b) What are the colors that represent your hero? Create a weaving in those colors.

    (c) Are you a hero to someone? Who might it be?

    (d) If you could do something heroic, what would it be?

(3) What do you do to pass the time when you are waiting? Demonstrate this in a movement. Create a "waiting" dance of all the responses you have together.

(4) Odysseus was gone for twenty years. What do you think he and Penelope said to each other when they first came together again?

(5) What do you think Odysseus looks like in Penelope's mind? (drawing)

(6) What do you think Penelope looks like in Odysseus' mind? (drawing)

(7) What are the sounds and smells of the kingdom of Ithaca? Create a soundscape/aroma-scape.

(8) Penelope created "home" for Odysseus. What does "home" mean to you? Create an open-format poem of the responses.

(9) Odysseus and Penelope's is a powerful love story. Is there a love story that you could tell from your own life?

(10) Young people don't know much about the lessons of a long-enduring love. What might you tell a young person about how to keep and tend love (of spouse, children, friends, etc.)?

(11) Penelope endured 108 suitors. What do you endure? Make a physical object that represents what you endure. It can be serious or silly.

(12) How/where do you think Penelope got the strength to endure twenty years alone?

(13) If this story took place today, do you think Penelope would do the same thing (wait twenty years)?

(14) How do you let people know they are welcome to your home? Make this into a dance.

(15) In ancient Greece, it was important to "welcome the stranger." What codes do we have about strangers?

(16) Penelope tested Odysseus to make sure it was him. How do you recognize people you love and who love you?

(17) A "chorus" in Greek drama is the voice of the community, commenting on the action of the play. If an audience watched your community, what is an action they might see? How might you comment on that action?

(18) Penelope's final words are, "If the gods really will grant us a happier old age, we'll be free from our trials at last." What do you think she meant?

(19) If Penelope could write a letter to Odysseus, what do you think she would say?

(20) How would she get her letter to him, so far away?

(21) Who makes "home" for you? How do they do this?

(22) Describe what home looks like. ("Home is" poem)

(23) What does it look like (physically) when you invite/greet someone into your home?

(24) What things make Luther Manor home? Who makes LM home? How?

(25) What advice do you have for Penelope?

(26) Penelope raised a son alone. What is some advice you would give Penelope about raising a son? What advice would you give Telemachus?

(27) Penelope would weave all day with her handmaidens. Can you make a weaving together with your friends that represents you individually and as a group?

APPENDIX 5. STORYTELLING AND PLAYWRITING SYLLABUS
The Penelope Project

SYLLABUS

SYLLABUS
THEATRE 359 Playwriting I
THEATRE 460 Storytelling
THEATRE 459 Playwriting II

Semester: Fall 2010

Credits: 3 credits per course (some of you are enrolled in both courses simultaneously—you will receive 6 credits for this experience)

Class Meeting Times: Tuesdays 2:00–4:45 p.m.

Final Celebration: 12/22/10 12:30–2:30 p.m.

Meeting Place: Mitchell 375/385 & Luther Manor, 4545 N. 92nd St., Milwaukee, WI 53225

Instructor for THEATRE 359 & 459: Dr. Anne Basting
    Contact Information: basting@uwm.edu, x2732
Instructor for THEATRE 460: Dr. Robin Mello
    Contact Information: rmello@uwm.edu, x6066

CATALOGUE DESCRIPTIONS

THEATRE 359: Playwriting process through in-class exercises, writing assignments, critical analysis, and discussion.

THEATRE 460: Development of skills to locate, analyze, and tell stories from multicultural sources and ranging from personal experience to myths and legends.

THEATRE 459: Advanced playwriting process through in-class exercises, writing assignments, critical analysis, and discussion.

359/459 COURSE LEARNING OUTCOMES

Students will be asked to:

(1) Collect imagination and memory-based stories from themselves and others from diverse perspectives
(2) Differentiate between "leading" and "facilitating" open group discussions
(3) Collaborate with a team to build an original, devised performance
(4) Analyze the structure and content of devised-theatre scripts
(5) Create original scenes
(6) Use proper play formatting

(7) Differentiate between subtext and text
(8) Create scenes using different styles of presentation (realistic, magical realism, and Brechtian meta-commentary)
(9) Interpret and analyze their own and others' writing and storytelling work

460 COURSE LEARNING OUTCOMES
Students will be asked to:
(1) Collect stories, memories, and imaginative discourse from themselves and others
(2) Tell, communicate, and perform stories
(3) Examine, collect, analyze, and reflect on stories from multicultural and/or diverse perspectives
(4) Create and participate in the storytelling art form
(5) Devise their own story-performance(s) and present them to others
(6) Demonstrate various techniques (such as vocalizations, gesture, dramatic structure, etc.) involved in creative performance-telling
(7) Interpret and analyze their own and others' storytelling work
(8) Participate in the creative process of making performance

GENERAL EDUCATION REQUIREMENT LEARNING (UWM GER)
Oral Communication (evaluated with Rubric posted online)
- Strengthening students' facility and familiarity in making language choices for dramatic presentations and theatrical communication.
- Developing storytelling delivery and performance skills.

The Arts (evaluated with Rubric posted online)
- Strengthening students' ability to craft story performances and devise theatrical presentations that integrate, incorporate, and reflect on multiple views and voices.
- Promoting students' ability to reflect on creative processes, especially those related to devising a community-based and issues-based performance.

DRESS CODE
There is a high professional standard at Luther Manor. Therefore, when students visit Luther Manor they are expected to wear clothing that is neat and clean. Students/visitors may *NOT* wear:
- Jeans
- T-shirts
- Miniskirts without long pants underneath
- Very high heels (they are unsafe in this situation)
- Flip-flops or open-toed sandals

- Ripped, skimpy, or revealing clothing (midriff must be covered)
- Low-cut shirts/pants that show most of breast/butt cleavage when you bend over (the aerial view is the thing to consider here)

Also . . .

- Piercings and tattoos should be displayed "modestly" (think as if you are going to a job interview, awards dinner, or religious service where respected elders are honored).
- Underwear should not be showing — this includes bras.
- Women should not go bra-less.

HIPAA

We are using the Standards for Privacy of Individually Identifiable Health Information, which is part of the Health Insurance Portability and Accountability Act of 1996 (HIPAA) as a guideline. Participants in this course may *NOT*:

- Disclose any patient information, directories of Luther Manor guests or clients, etc.
- Disclose private health information to people who are not in this class. If you want to ask questions or discuss perceptions, use our private online course website — it is private and not subject to outside access.
- Disclose or discuss details about the medical condition of people at Luther Manor outside this research or class project. This includes social networking and socializing in general.

We've posted the HIPAA law at our online course site. HIPAA does allow all of us to talk about conditions such as dementia in general ways and through chat it calls "incidental" disclosure for purposes of education/research. We have obtained IRB permission to do research and will discuss this at length in class as well.

PENELOPE PROJECT COURSES GENERAL GUIDELINES

This is going to be a great project, but it might kick up some surprising feelings for you. If you are having any kinds of issues with class at all, please contact Anne or Robin in any of our communication modes — email, phone, even come by the office. *We are here to talk it through.*

- The focus of the course is primarily on active participation: *we are all learning and we are all teaching.*
- This course requires a commitment of time and some travel (because it is about experiencing the community around us instead of a classroom-based experience).
- Expect to work outside of class as well as during class time.
- Expect to check the online site and calendar frequently so you know what is going on ahead of time.

- Luther Manor has a dress code: it is clearly explained in the syllabus. Be familiar with it. Follow it.
- In class and in sessions during discussions and story sharing, use "I" statements: speak for yourself.
- Encourage questions and sharing of feelings, perspectives, beliefs, and ideas. Try things out first before accepting or rejecting.
- Acknowledge viewpoints other than your own as valid. Remember, you don't have to *agree* with people to acknowledge others' ideas and perspectives.
- Avoid making other people tokens. (Example: Although Robin is a middle-aged woman, she can't necessarily speak for *all* middle-aged women. . . . You get the idea.)
- Disagree and challenge respectfully.
- Respect and support each other as creative and successful.
- Have fun, enjoy, play, and explore your creative self.
- *Spend the time you need to really do the work well, thoroughly, and completely. Make this a learning experience that works for you.*
- Respect the confidentiality of all participants; the classroom needs to be a safe space. THIS MEANS THAT YOU CAN'T REPORT ANECDOTES FROM THE COURSE WORK ON FACEBOOK, LINKEDIN, OR OTHER SOCIAL NETWORK SYSTEMS. Beware of gossiping—especially as a tweet or blog.
- Check in to the online course site frequently. Use the resources there.
- Attempt to "unpack" and examine your assumptions and biases on a regular basis. Attempt to identify the assumptions and biases of others.
- It's OK to let us know if you feel disrespected, unheard, or upset. Doing so (use the I statement) is often the best response to these feelings.
- It's OK to call for a moment of silence or request a slower pace.
- It is also OK to ask for a standing ovation.

READINGS

Chapter 1: "What Are Myths?"	From *A Short History of Myth* by Karen Armstrong (e-reserve)
Chapter 2: "Home"	From *Six Myths of Our Time* by Marina Warner (e-reserve)
"Artists in Action"	In *American Theatre Magazine*, summer 2010 (e-reserve)
"The End of the Iliad"	From *Dateline: Troy* by Paul Fleishman (e-reserve)
Fires in the Mirror	Film on reserve in media library
Vagina Monologues	Film on reserve in media library
O Brother, Where Art Thou?	Film on reserve in media library
My Trip to Al-Qaeda	Airing on HBO 9/7/10 or 9/11/10

Art Care	By Anne Basting (e-reserve)
Chapter 6: Storytelling	From *Local Acts* by Jan Cohen-Cruz (e-reserve)
Chapter 7: Structures	From *Local Acts* by Jan Cohen-Cruz (e-reserve)
Chapter 1: Starting Points	From *Playbuilding* by Errol Bray (e-reserve)

CALENDAR

Date/Place	Activities	What Is Due?
9/7 On campus	• Introduce ourselves • Look over syllabus • Warm-up • Story card / universal themes • Introduce research project • Consent forms • Logistics • HIPAA: role-play simulation • Discuss reading • Reviewing what is due next week	• Read & look at the online course site • Have syllabus (hard copy) as a ticket to the class. • Completed first survey online • Completed all parts of the first assignment including the readings and be ready to discuss
9/14 On campus	• Meet/greet • Story tag • Singing in the stairway • Review logistics • Reminder about the auditions • I AM poems—constructing a voice • Devising step #1: knowing your own story • Devising step #2: listening • Devising step #3: themes & perspectives • Elder circle • Review story collection/gathering • Review ethics • Introduction and discussion about the final celebration • Group dynamics and assigned jobs, etc.	• Creative responses to reading • Bring a hard copy of "How to Interview a Stone Wall" to class (it is your ticket) • Almost EVERYONE will have questions about this course; bring them with you
9/21 On campus	• Guest: Dr. Andrew Porter • "How to Interview a Stone Wall"— simulations • Group devising groups assigned • Dramaturgical notes • Reading • Discussion • Person-centered inquiry • Practicing what you will do at Luther Manor	• Index cards due: they are your ticket to class • Did you do any of the extra-credit assignments? If so, be ready to share your impressions • Today we will be deciding on group membership for final performances • AFTER THE CLASS IS COMPLETE you will be posting your poem online
9/28 On campus	• Telling the *Odyssey* in under 10 minutes • Hero and heroine life-cycle process exploration • Beth M. comes to visit • Questions for Beth Meyer-Arnold	• Questions posted online • Questions printed out is your ticket to class • Protocols due by the 2nd of Oct.!!! That means that your group should be meeting outside of class
10/5 @ Luther Manor	• Sessions at Luther Manor	• Protocols posted online • Ensure that you are set with any technology or items you need • Bring writing implements and paper, laptops, or other technologies, etc. with you to Luther Manor • Remember there is a dress code

Date/Place	Activities	What Is Due?
10/12 @ Luther Manor FRIDAY 10/14	• Sessions at Luther Manor • Auditions with Sojourn Theatre Co. @ Theatre Basement Rehearsal Rooms 6 and 7	• We are looking forward to seeing you there
10/19 On campus	• Check-in with groups • Check-in as a class community • Meet and discuss the work with Sojourn visiting artists	• Reading responses posted online • Ensure that you are meeting with your group outside of class time
10/26 @ Luther Manor	• Sessions at Luther Manor	
11/2 @ Luther Manor	• Sessions at Luther Manor	
11/9 On campus	• Midterm check-in • Coding—what does this all mean? • Playwriting students meet with Anne • Storytellers work on games with Robin	• Group check-in posted online • Transcripts have been posted for each group (check the assignment requirements for details) • Each student in this class should have a copy of at least one transcript to work on in class • Coding procedures handout is your ticket to class
11/16 @ Luther Manor	• Sessions at Luther Manor	• Reminder: you and your group should be meeting outside of class in order to practice, hone, and edit the final presentation and script
11/23 No class meeting scheduled	• Take an early turkey break and check-in online—we will not be meeting officially at Luther Manor or on campus	• We suggest that you take this time to catch up on stuff, read, and enjoy the short holiday break
11/30 On campus	• Final presentation check-in • Work in class on building your presentation • Show and tell: groups show what they've been working on • Group juggling / juggling as metaphor • Research survey (given in class)	• Keep honing the final presentation and final script
12/7 @ Luther Manor	• This is the final visit before our final celebration; wrap things up and rehearse.	
12/14 @ Luther Manor	• This is our celebration day!	• Presentations @ Luther Manor
12/16 @ Luther Manor	• We meet in the Welcome Area to debrief, wrap-up, evaluate, and reflect	• Final scripts are due in the drop-box online • Final surveys due

APPENDIX 6. A NOTE ON THE PROGRAM EVALUATION
Robin Mello

The program evaluation that informs the chapter "What Did the Research Tell Us?" in part five is primarily qualitative in nature and concentrated on the efficacy and impact of Penelope. It is a summative review of how the project evolved, created meaningful work, and met its goals. The report also addresses the evolution of the project and its effect on participants' learning and quality of life.

The program evaluation is grounded in the blended methodologies of narrative inquiry, arts-based action research, and utilization assessment — with qualitative inquiry as its primary framework. The project's intent in pursuing a qualitative perspective was to capture a nuanced and multifaceted picture of its many and varied enterprises. Qualitative inquiry provides opportunities for deep iterative analysis and includes various and multiple perspectives that are held by diverse constituencies.

The validity of the research is ensured through the use of data triangulation — that is, examination and collection of multiple data points with an emphasis on the impressions and reactions of constituents. Triangulation was also used in vetting the information within this report — it was presented as a draft to a number of people who had an official interest in learning about the Penelope Project (PP) outcomes. Their input helped shape and modify the information in this report.

An impartial observer did not write this report. The primary evaluator (Mello) is an "insider." Therefore, this evaluation depends significantly on action research perspectives, which allowed this researcher to engage in evaluation activities before, during, and after participating in performance-related work, storytelling sessions, and direct instruction. She also utilized the concept of "critical friend,"[1] a concept that is used to promote constructive critique when collecting and analyzing evaluation data. Further, during the report-writing year, Mello took a "back seat" to major PP initiatives, acting in a role that was primarily observational.

THEORETICAL VALIDITY AND PERSPECTIVES

The principal investigators who collaborated in the PP have all published or produced creative and scholarly work relating to its subject/context. Further, these authors and artists base their works on the assumption that participating in creative work and artistic exploration can foster engaged relationships and invigorated perspectives toward society. It is not surprising, then, to find that one of the primary threads that runs through all their works is a deep understanding for, application of, and compassionate engagement with respect for elders with dementia. As one of the project's leaders noted:

There are banners hung on the outside of schools that say, "High expectations start here." We need to hang those on care facilities. These can be places to live, learn, grow, and thrive. . . . I want people to feel that. I want people to think that. I want people to fight for that and make it happen.

The program evaluation acknowledges these perspectives and works within it. It is predicated on the idea that creativity and compassion are fundamental to the human condition.

DESCRIPTIVE VALIDITY AND METHOD

Data sources for the program evaluation include program documents, grant narratives, surveys, evaluation questionnaires, video recordings of activities and meetings, documentary film footage, emails and phone conversations, participant observations, site visits, focus groups, and in-depth interviews.

PARTICIPANTS

The following constituent groups were sampled and contacted for this evaluation:
- 7 LM resident chorus members
- All cast and crew members
- 5 Sojourn Theatre company members
- 7 designer, director, and management personnel
- 6 UWM student researchers
- 26 (all) UWM 460, 359, and 459 students
- 4 UWM instructors
- 32 percent of audience members
- 10 LM administrators / staff members / facilitators
- 7 think-tank participants
- 3 LM volunteers
- 2 UWM administrators
- 2 UWM alumni

QUESTIONS

Areas of inquiry answered by the program evaluation are as follows:
(1) The scope and context of the project: how the PP evolved and developed.
(2) The extent to which the PP succeeded in meeting its stated outcomes and goals.
(3) The impact of the PP program on participants.
(4) Suggestions for models for future programming, including sustainability and replication.

NOTES

1. Mello, R. 2005. "Close Up and Personal: The Effect of a Researcher's Relationship on an Educational Program Evaluation." *Teachers College Record* 107 (11): 1056–67.

APPENDIX 7. FUNDING PARTNERS
(IN ALPHABETICAL ORDER)

The American Association of Homes and Services for the Aging (AAHSA)
(now called Leading Age)
Lead: Beth Meyer-Arnold, Luther Manor
AAHSA contributed in-kind dissemination support.

The Brookdale Foundation ($17,000)
Lead: Anne Basting, UWM's Center on Age & Community (CAC)
The Brookdale Foundation approved a CAC request for re-appropriation of unspent
 funds left from a grant program designed to support an artist residency for
 people with dementia.

The Doris Duke Charitable Trust and the Rockefeller Foundation's
Multi-Arts Production Fund (MAP) ($35,000)
Lead: Michael Rohd, Sojourn Theatre
MAP funds were awarded to support the conceptual development, shaping, and
 sharing of a professional-quality, site-specific performance at Luther Manor and
 to use this production to create a replicable arts-based engagement model for
 future use in educational and community settings.

Faye McBeath Foundation ($15,000)
Co-leads: Anne Basting, UWM's CAC; Robin Mello, UWM Department of Theatre
McBeath awarded a grant to establish an ongoing service-learning model for UWM
 students to work with Milwaukee long-term care facilities, including adult day,
 assisted living, and skilled nursing centers.

The Forest County Potawatomi Community Foundation (FCPCP) ($10,000)
Lead: Beth Meyer-Arnold, Luther Manor
Penelope was a strong fit with FCPCP's mission to strengthen communities and
 provide examples of responsible citizenship. Our focus on intergenerational
 storytelling and the power of myth was another factor for receiving this FCPCP
 award.

The Helen Bader Foundation (HBF) ($20,000)
Lead: Anne Basting, UWM's CAC
Existing monies that support CAC core programs and product development were
 used to create a model program, support Meyer-Arnold as consultant, and
 document the project on film.

Imagining America
Lead: Anne Basting, UWM's CAC
Indirect support for dissemination, particularly in association with the workshop
(Using the Arts and Humanities in Community Health) held in conjunction
with the final performance of *Finding Penelope*.

Luther Manor Health Care Center and Adult Day Services
Lead: Beth Meyer-Arnold, Luther Manor
In-kind contributions for management of the project and use of the Luther Manor
van for transportation.

Picker Institute ($24,000)
Lead: Anne Basting, UWM's CAC
Direct support of the book-planning retreat.

Sojourn Theatre
Lead: Michael Rohd, Artistic Director
Sojourn Theatre supported the project by providing in-kind contributions,
administrative oversight, and artistic vision.

Support for Undergraduate Research Fellows Program (SURF) ($3,000)
Co-leads: Anne Basting, UWM; Robin Mello, UWM
Funds provided to UWM undergraduate students for dramaturgical research.

The United Lutheran Program for the Aging, Inc. (ULPA)
Lead: Beth Meyer-Arnold, Luther Manor
ULPA contributed direct support as well as in-kind and dissemination support.

UWM Department of Theatre
Co-leads: Anne Basting and Robin Mello
Visiting-artist funds; in-kind donation for faculty load and management of the
project; and use of classrooms, materials, supplies, and marketing were provided
to Penelope from the department.

UWM's Center on Age & Community
Lead: Anne Basting, Director
Support for management of the project.

Wisconsin Arts Board: Artist and Community Collaborations Grant (A&CC)
($4,500)
Lead: Beth Meyer-Arnold, Luther Manor
A&CC funds supported playwright Anne Basting's developmental work on the
project.

Wisconsin Humanities Council: Major Grant (WHC) ($10,000)
Lead: Beth Meyer-Arnold, Luther Manor
The grant specified using monies to promote "the power of the humanities to catalyze growth in both individuals and communities" and supported the early developmental work of Anne Basting, Robin Mello, and classicist Andrew Porter.

The Wisconsin Representatives of Activity Professionals (WRAP) ($2,000)
Lead: Anne Basting, UWM's CAC
WRAP provided direct support as well as in-kind and dissemination support.

APPENDIX 8. SURVEY QUESTIONS

This survey was provided by Susan McFadden (PhD) and adapted from the Dementia Attitudes Scale validated by Melissa O'Connor and Susan McFadden.

The following statements were presented with a five-point Likert scale (strongly disagree; disagree; neither agree nor disagree; agree; strongly agree):

(1) I enjoy being around old people.
(2) I like to go visit my older relatives.
(3) I enjoy talking with old people.
(4) I feel very comfortable when I am around an old person.
(5) I enjoy doing things for old people.
(6) I fear it will be very hard for me to find contentment in old age.
(7) I will have plenty to occupy my time when I am old.
(8) I expect to feel good about life when I am old.
(9) I believe that I will be able to do most things for myself when I am old.
(10) I have never lied about my age in order to appear younger.
(11) It doesn't bother me at all to imagine myself as being old.
(12) I have never dreaded the day I would look in the mirror and see gray hairs.
(13) I have never dreaded looking old.
(14) When I look in the mirror it bothers me to see how my looks have changed with age.
(15) I fear that when I am old all my friends will be gone.
(16) The older I become, the more I worry about my health.
(17) I get nervous when I think about someone else making decisions for me when I am old.
(18) I worry that people will ignore me when I am old.
(19) I am afraid that there will be no meaning in life when I am old.
(20) It is rewarding to work with people who have Alzheimer's (Alz.) disease or dementia.
(21) People with Alz. disease or dementia can be creative.
(22) I am afraid of people with Alz. disease or dementia.
(23) I am comfortable being around people with Alz. disease or dementia.
(24) I am not very familiar with Alz. disease or dementia.
(25) It is possible to enjoy interacting with people with Alz. disease or dementia.
(26) I feel relaxed around people with Alz. disease or dementia.
(27) People with Alz. disease or dementia can enjoy life.

(28) I cannot imagine taking care of someone with Alz. disease or dementia.

(29) We can do a lot now to improve the lives of people with Alz. disease or dementia.

(30) People with Alz. disease or dementia can feel when others are kind to them.

Anne Basting is an educator, artist, and scholar focusing on creative community engagement. She was founding director of University of Wisconsin–Milwaukee's Center on Age & Community from 2003 to 2013. Basting is currently professor of theatre in the Peck School of the Arts at UWM, and founder and president of the nonprofit TimeSlips Creative Storytelling (www.timeslips.org). She wrote the script for *Finding Penelope* and managed the overall Penelope Project.

Jan Cohen-Cruz is a scholar, practitioner, and teacher of grassroots, socially grounded, and activist art. She is author of *Engaging Performance: Theatre as Call and Response* and *Local Acts: Community-Based Performance in the US*; she edited *Radical Street Performance*; and, with Mady Schutzman, she coedited *Playing Boal: Theatre, Therapy, Activism* and *A Boal Companion: Dialogues on Theatre and Cultural Politics*. She is University Professor at Syracuse University.

Daniel Jake Cohen is an actor and teaching artist based in Oakland. Prior to working on the Penelope Project, Jake worked on Sojourn Theatre's 2010 production *On the Table*. He is currently pursuing his MA in Montessori early childhood education at St. Mary's College of California. Cohen helped develop and perform *Finding Penelope*.

Leonard Cruz holds an MFA in performance/choreography and a PhD in urban education from the University of Wisconsin–Milwaukee. As a professional dancer, Cruz performed with Robert Wilson, with Pina Bausch, and for five years with Bill T. Jones / Arne Zane. Cruz choreographed *Finding Penelope*.

Angela Fingard is a theatre artist and mental health educator. As a returning student in the UWM Department of Theatre, Fingard was part of the Storytelling class that facilitated creative discussions as Luther Manor, and then worked as assistant director of *Finding Penelope*.

Jolene Hansen has volunteered at Luther Manor for over twenty years. A former English teacher, Hansen led writing workshops as part of the Penelope Project. She is author of *I Bring Daffodils*, a series of essays about her experiences with creative engagement in adult day settings.

Joyce Heinrich is a resident at Luther Manor who performed in *Finding Penelope*. Heinrich says, "The older I get, the more I look forward to each new day. At eighty-five, I love to travel, try new things, brush up on my writing and storytelling, and serve others through church activities."

Robin Mello is a professional storyteller, certified special education teacher, and narrative scholar who has toured internationally as a teller of tales and teaching-artist for over twenty years. Robin holds a PhD from Leslie University. She has published articles in *The Educational Forum, Journal of Qualitative Research*, and *The International Journal of Arts in Education*, to name a few. Currently she teaches storytelling as well as theatre methods and fieldwork, and she directs the K-12 Theatre Education at UWM. Robin performed in, taught classes for, and led the program evaluation for the Penelope Project.

Beth Meyer-Arnold was director of Adult Day and Community Services at Luther Manor for twenty-five years, where she pioneered person-centered care in both programming and environmental design. With Lyn Geboy, Meyer-Arnold is author of *Person-Centered Care in Practice: Tools for Transformation* (Attainment Co.). She is a principal with Cygnet Innovations Group LLC.

Ellie Rose is a visual artist and dementia care specialist. Her arts-engagement strategies focus on brain exercise, arts education, and creative enlightenment for people living with cognitive impairments.

Michael Rohd is founding artistic director of Sojourn Theatre, on faculty at Northwestern University, and author of the widely translated book *Theatre for Community, Conflict, and Dialogue*. His work focuses on social practice, civic practice, and capacity-building projects through collaboratively designed arts-based event, engagement, and participation strategies. He leads the Center for Performance and Civic Practice and is the 2013–2016 Doris Duke artist-in-residence at Chicago's Lookingglass Theatre Company.

Maureen Towey directs live performance events. She works as a creative director for musicians such as Arcade Fire and Ray LaMontagne. She has been recognized as an AOL/PBS MAKER, a Princess Grace fellow, a TCG Leadership U Fellow, and a Fulbright scholar in South Africa. She is an ensemble member of Sojourn Theatre and a graduate of Northwestern University.

Rusty Tym is a resident at Luther Manor. Says Tym: "Life just keeps getting better! At seventy-six, thanks to *Finding Penelope*, I'm directing plays, learning new writing concepts, enjoying all I'm doing, and facing life with the hope of being of service toward the most interesting people in the world: those I come in contact with."

Julie Voigts is an alum of the UWM Department of Theatre. She worked as the liaison to Luther Manor for UWM during the Penelope Project and was later hired by Luther Manor as a person-centered care specialist.

Nikki Zaleski is the education and arts justice manager for the Illinois Caucus for Adolescent Health (ICAH), where she designs participatory theatre experiences about sexual health and sexual violence with the FYI Performance Cadre. Nikki is an artistic associate for Sojourn Theatre, is a company member of Erasing the Distance, and has directed performances for Redmoon Theater, Northwestern University, Ag47, and Urban Gateways. She holds a BA in performance studies and gender studies from Northwestern and an MA in interdisciplinary studies from DePaul University.